OLD IS NOT A FOUR-LETTER WORD

SHEILA ROBERTS

CONTENTS

Author's Note 5
Preface: New Beginnings 7

1. Famous Third Act Successes 11
2. Success in Their Corner of the World 19
3. Bible Stories for Seniors 37
4. Older, Wiser, And Willing to Work 45
5. To Your Health 57
6. What Now, My Love? Lifestyle Changes and Challenges 84
7. Life After Death: Coping With Loss 101
8. Here's Looking at You... Still 113
9. Not Limited by a Limited Income 125
10. Boomer Beware 139
11. Before the Curtain is Pulled 151
12. Encouraging Words 164

Acknowledgments 169

AUTHOR'S NOTE

Statistics I've quoted and information I've shared in this book were, to my knowledge, accurate at the time of the writing. As we know, however, the cost of living goes up, new research appears, and statistics change. On all important life matters, please always consult an expert in the field. This book is an overview and if you are wanting to know more about any of the topics discussed I would encourage you to research them further and read the books I've mentioned. I found all of them to be excellent reading.

PREFACE: NEW BEGINNINGS

Allow me to start by saying I'm no expert. Not a doctor, not an elder law attorney, not a financial planner. Just someone like you, trying to live this final part of my life as successfully as I can. (Which is why I'm including thoughts and advice from others right along with my own. Together we can figure this stuff out!) Like you, I've waved good-bye to middle-age and stepped over the threshold into what is often referred to as old age.

Many of us prefer to think of this phase of life as our golden years or refer to ourselves as senior citizens or seasoned citizens. Whatever we call it, a lot of us have mixed feelings about where we are now. I know I do. I'm thankful for the wisdom I've acquired and I love being able to afford to do some of the things I couldn't when my husband and I were younger and raising a family. But I'm not fond of the wrinkles or the aches and pains that have started surfacing. Are you feeling the same way?

Let me share a couple of anecdotes with you. Not to depress you, I promise. I'm only starting out by making a point. Hang in there with me because, like this book, your story isn't over yet.

A few years ago, a friend who had hit her sixties lamented, "We're invisible. Nobody sees us." I was surprised by her comment because this woman is beautiful. Who wouldn't notice her? I thought she was delirious and said so. I couldn't even relate. I certainly didn't feel like I was being ignored. Perhaps that was because I've always been a bit of a spotlight hog. I'm still a working writer and I make appearances and do book signings, which pretty much forces people to pay attention to me.

Recently, however, I realized that I'm not exactly turning heads. But so what? I can still turn my husband's head. He happens to like this older woman.

Still, my friend's words stuck with me. Were we men and women "of a certain age" invisible?

A few Christmases back I noticed something unsettling. I was at the big Christmas Eve gathering with my extended family, seated at the same table as one of the grandmas, a very sweet older woman, pushing ninety. I noticed that people (including myself) talked with her, but the conversations were brief. They chatted a moment and then moved on to invest more conversational energy in younger family members and other activities. It occurred to me that, even though she was present, she hadn't been brought in to be a vital part of what was going on. Everyone else was in the game, but she was left sitting on the sidelines. All the other relatives her age were now dead; she was the last one of her generation left. Somehow, her sitting at the outside edges of the family circle didn't seem right. Looking back on that day, I can't help but wish that we'd all gathered around her, listened as she recounted her experiences and the lessons she'd learned over the years, and encouraged her to reminisce about Christmases past.

I've come to realize how important it is to spend time with those who are older than us. They're the keepers of the family history. They've experienced hard times and survived. We can learn so much from them. With age comes wisdom, and because of that older people have their own unique place in the scheme of things. Sometimes it can be difficult to find that place here in America as our culture doesn't always acknowledge this fact. We worship youth. And I guess that's the point I'm trying to make. The western world doesn't make aging easy.

But just because our culture worships youth, we don't have to join in. There's a great verse in the Bible that tells us not to conform to this world's standards but to let God transform our minds to a better way of thinking.[1] Western culture tells us that we must be forever young and good looking. Sexy! In God's culture we're valuable no matter what we look like, no matter our age. (I'll give you some examples of this later.)

No matter what your religious belief system, I hope you'll be able to appreciate the universal truth underlying some of the examples I'll use. I suspect we can agree on the basic principle that we all have value, whatever our age. I much prefer that way of thinking to the one that says, "Throw Grandma off the bus. She's just taking up space." Don't you?

Yes, my dewy days are over. The dew has long since died on this little rose. However, that doesn't mean I can't still bloom, that I can't do worthwhile things and enjoy life. The same goes for you!

By this time of life we have lived much, seen much, and learned much. Because of that we have much to offer. As long as we're breathing and our minds are still working we have a purpose for being here. Old is not the same as dead. Old is wise, old is valuable. Old is still needed. Like the ads in the classifieds say, "Experience Wanted."

This may be our third act, but the play is not over yet and there is still a part for each of us. Old is not a four-letter word.

1. "Do not conform to the pattern of this world, but be transformed by the renewing of your mind..." Romans 2:12, New International Version, Copyright 1984.

1. FAMOUS THIRD ACT SUCCESSES

The third act in a play is when everything comes together. It can be the same with our lives. This final phase can be one of satisfaction and success, and I'd like to offer up as examples several people who are a good example of how to write a great third act. Let's kick things off by talking about ones who have made an impression on the world stage.

Laura Ingalls Wilder

Born in 1867 into a pioneer family, this woman grew up homesteading in Wisconsin, Missouri, Kansas, Minnesota and the Dakotas. She did a brief stint as a school teacher, then married and spent the bulk of her life farming and raising her family. She didn't take up writing until around 1910. She couldn't find a publisher for her first book, a memoir titled *Pioneer Girl*, so she rewrote it and titled it *Little House in the Big Woods*. This became the first book in her famous children's series, and she was sixty-five when it was first published. (Some sources say sixty-four – either way, she was not young.) She continued writing, and the last of her books came out when she was seventy-six years old.

. . .

Grandma Moses

Anna Mary Moses, who later became known as Grandma Moses, was born in 1860. She began to paint at the age of seventy-eight. In her autobiography she says she started painting "for pleasure, to keep busy and to pass the time away..." [1] Obviously, her folksy paintings had made an impression on her friends because one of them suggested that she show some of them at the local drug store in Hoosick Falls, where she lived.

An art collector passing through bought them and wanted to know who had painted them. Oh, and by the way, he wanted ten more. She pulled together ten paintings for him (making her count by actually cutting one in half), and he asked her to paint more. He took her paintings to New York to show in galleries and three of them wound up in a Museum of Modern Art exhibition. After that, it was on to an exclusive art gallery. This was followed by a Thanksgiving exhibition at Gimbels' auditorium. After that came radio appearances, dinner with the Women's National Press Club, honorary doctoral degrees, and tea with the First Lady. Governor Nelson Rockefeller named the day of her hundredth birthday Grandma Moses Day. Her paintings appeared on everything from greeting cards to fabrics.[2] Not bad for a woman who was self-taught and didn't get around to devoting herself to her art until she was in her seventies. What strikes me most as I read about this woman was that she was willing to go through any door that opened. Are you? Am I? I hope so!

Helen Hooven Santmyer

Even before she became famous Helen was no slouch. She was a teacher, served as dean of women and head of the English Department at Cedarville College in Ohio, and then became a reference librarian in the Dayton and Montgomery County Public Library after her retirement. But she was known for her novel *And the Ladies of the Club*, which was published when she was in her eighties. This was a project she had worked on for years. In its first publication with a small press the book only sold a few hundred copies. But word of mouth brought her to the attention of a Los Angeles producer, and from there it found its way to the prestigious William Morris Agency in New York. William Morris sold it to G.P. Putnam's Sons and it became a hit.[3] It was a Book of the Month Club selection, and a New York Times #1 bestseller – achievements most authors only dream of.

Reading this woman's story, I was struck, not only by the fact that fame finally found her when she was eighty-seven, but also by her persistence. She continued to work at a story she believed in. She persevered, putting that story out there, and eventually her work paid off.

Fauja Singh

As of this writing, Fauja Singh holds the record for being the oldest marathon runner in the world. Nicknamed the Turbaned Tornado, he took up running at eighty-nine. Fame found him when he completed a full 26.2-mile marathon in six hours and fifty-four minutes. (I could do that... maybe in six days and fifty-four minutes!) Last I read he was still running at one-hundred six.[4]

How did he get started? After raising his family, he and his wife settled in to enjoy their golden years and visit their children, who were living abroad. That ended when he was eighty-one with the death of his wife. Two years later his son, who had been caring for him after the death of his wife, was killed in a construction accident. Still grieving, he eventually moved to London to stay with another son. His life changed for the better the day he heard an anchor on a TV news show inviting people to take part in the upcoming London Marathon. Fauja accepted that invitation. He got a coach, trained, and ran the marathon.

At one hundred one he ran the London Marathon in seven

hours and forty-nine minutes. This man proved you don't have to be a twenty-something football star to get ad campaign contracts. He was signed by Adidas for its "Nothing is Impossible" ad campaign and was also seen running in a Ford commercial.

Check him out on Youtube and Facebook. Maybe after seeing him you'll want to put on your running shoes, too.

Diana Nyad

At the age of sixty-four Diana Nyad finally made a dream that she'd had since she was eight years old come true. After four tries over thirty-five years, she finally became the first person to swim from Florida to Cuba without a protective shark cage. (Every time I read this I can't help but hear the music from *Jaws* playing in my head.) I love her quote regarding late life success: "One is we should never, ever give up. Two is you are never are too old to chase your dreams."[5]

Evelyn Williams

This lady is a great example of chasing her dreams at a time in life when many people probably would find what she did to be ridiculous. If you don't hang out a lot on Facebook or happen to live in Ireland, her name may not be familiar to you. If that's the case, do a quick search and you'll see this eighty-two-year old woman wowing the judges on Ireland's TV talent show, *Ireland's Got Talent*. Her rendition of "Send in the Clowns" earned her the golden buzzer and she went on to make the semi-finals. Go Evelyn!

Dorothy Davenhill Hirsch

This woman never stopped doing interesting things. Poke around on the internet and you'll find she traveled throughout her life and was the quintessential volunteer. She didn't let a little detail like age stop her from traveling and she made it into the Guinness Book of World Records at eighty-nine, becoming the oldest person to go to the North Pole.

Let's move further back in history.

Benjamin Franklin

Famous for the part he played in the American revolution and drafting our constitution, Benjamin Franklin was also a scientist and inventor. He was well into his golden years when he made bifocal glasses stylish.[6]

Louis Pasteur

Louis Pasteur gave the first injection against rabies to a human when he was sixty-three.[7] For a long time, many of us in the United States were retired by this age.

Peter Roget

This man published the thesaurus we writers all love so much and depend on to enlarge our vocabulary. He was seventy-three when he did this, and he oversaw every update until he died at the age of ninety.[8] He was forced to retire from the Royal Society, London's association of esteemed scientists when he neared seventy to make way for the younger generation. (I wonder how many of them made as great or lasting contribution to the world.)

No Room on Stage?

Don't you find it interesting that, even generations ago, the young were anxious to push the old out of the way so they could have their time on stage? Well, folks, it's a big stage and there's room for all of us.

Many of my writing pals are no longer young, but they're still going strong and refuse to let anyone set a cut-off date for their careers. Take for example romance writer, Carolyn Brown. As of this writing Carolyn is sixty-nine and, as she says, is "starin' seventy in the face and not mindin' it since the alternative doesn't look real good." Retirement is the farthest thing from her mind. She plans to retire only if the voices in her head stop talking to her. (This is writer speak for "If I can't think up any new characters.") Her advice is to work as long as you can. "My uncle retired on Friday and dropped dead with a heart attack on Sunday. I'm going to produce books as long as I have a mind and fingers to type," she says. "And when I go, it's going to be in the small window of opportunity between my last contract and the one I'm about to sign, so I go out with everything finished and in to the editors."

Sometimes it can feel like we've been toiling away for years without seeing the results we want. If that's the case with you, don't give up. We all plant in different fields and in different ways and some crops take a while to grow. I always laugh at my friend Debbie Macomber's quip that it took her twenty years to become an overnight success.

Maybe your big moment is right around the corner, like Paul Cézanne, who had his first solo art exhibition at the age of fifty-six.[9] Then there's Nelson Mandela, who was elected president of South Africa at seventy-five.[10]

Don't drop the curtain on your life story too soon. Get out there and be and do. You never know what future fulfillment or success awaits you in your third act.

1. Grandma Moses, *Grandma Moses, My Life's History,* edit. by Otto Kallir, (Harper & Brothers, 1948).

2. Judith Stein, "The White-Haired Girl: A Feminist Reading," in

Grandma Moses in the 21st Century, (New Haven, Yale University Press, 2001), pp. 48 – 63.

3. Herbert Mitgang, *Helen Hooven Santmyer*, obituary, *The New York Times*, (February 22, 1986).

4. "106 Year Fauja Singh to Start Birmingham Marathon," October 4, 2017. https://www.greatrun.org/news-and-media/news/106-year-old-fauja-singh-to-start-birmingham-marathon#yjsAFA5SWwvuQMIq.97

5. Matt Pearce, "Diana Nyad after Swim: 'You're Never Too Old to Chase Your Dreams,'" *Los Angeles Times*, September 2, 2013.
https://www.latimes.com/nation/nationnow/la-na-nn-diana-nyad-cuba-florida-remarks-20130902-story.html

6. Timetoast.com: Benjamin Franklin: Inventor Timeline, Copyright 2007 – 2019. https://www.timetoast.com/timelines/benjamin-franklin-inventor

7. Sciencehistory.org: Louis Pasteur, Copyright 2019.
https://www.sciencehistory.org/historical-profile/louis-pasteur

8. Molly Edmonds and Becky Striepe, "Peter Mark Roget Compiles Thesaurus," *10 Famous Accomplishments Made Late in Life*, Copyright 2019. https://health.howstuffworks.com/wellness/

aging/senior-health-lifestyle/5-famous-accomplishments-made-late-in-life7.htm

9. Artble.com: Paul Cezanne, Copyright 2019. https://www.artble.com/artists/paul_cezanne

10. Howstuffworks.com: “Nelson Mandela Becomes President of South Africa,” Copyright 2019. https://health.howstuffworks.com/wellness/aging/senior-health-lifestyle/5-famous-accomplishments-made-late-in-life3.htm

2. SUCCESS IN THEIR CORNER OF THE WORLD

In the previous chapter I shared several stories of people who continued to be productive later in life, many actually hitting their stride after so-called retirement age. In this chapter I'd like to talk about some seniors who, while not world famous, have made a difference in their corner of the world and are still enjoying rewarding pursuits. Let me start with a man I admired hugely, my oldest brother.

BEN MOYLE

When he died at the age of eighty-two it was a huge loss, not only for our family but for his whole community. Brother Ben was a busy guy. He was coaching basketball, taking voice lessons and entering vocal competitions along with college students young enough to be his grandkids right up until the day a stroke took him down. He was active in his church and the heart of, not only his immediate family, but our entire extended family.

When someone dies at an advanced age, the attendance at the memorial service can be a little sparse. Not so with Ben. The celebration of his life was held in a church that probably seated a couple hundred people and it was packed. The service lasted for two hours. The first half hour was a message taken from his final words of advice to his family. The rest of the time people stood and shared their memories. I lost count of how many people recounted how he'd helped them in one way or another.

All this for a man who worked a simple job in a warehouse. Smart enough to run a company, he never wanted the pressure and was happy to work a job that kept him in the background rather than the forefront. He never held office, never headed a corporation, never got a chance to become that famous singer he could have been. My brother wasn't famous, just important to many people.

Ben was wired to help others, and even when his family was young he was always doing something for someone – helping a neighbor move, taking the neighborhood kids to the nearest ball field and hitting balls to them, roofing someone's house – whatever you needed, he was there. He had five children but my niece said none of them ever felt cheated, never felt as though Ben didn't have time for them. He managed to make each of them feel special.

And he continued to make people feel special, even more so after he retired. In fact, retirement set my brother free to really get busy. We sold my mother's house in the city and moved her to the family property on a small island in the Pacific Northwest, putting her in a modular home between our houses and his. Not a day went by when he didn't bring her lunch and dinner. I often offered to take a meal but the only time I was allowed was when my brother and sis-in-law, Marliss, went out of town.

Taking care of Mom was just the beginning. At an age when many of his friends were ready to relax and enjoy life, one of my nephews and his three daughters moved in with Ben and suddenly, once again, his life was full with school schedules and chauffeuring.

The last granddaughter left the nest only a year before my brother died. He didn't have time for empty nest syndrome though. He was too busy coaching girls' basketball. He also coached his grandson's basketball team. The day he had his stroke he'd had a voice lesson scheduled and a game to coach. I'm surprised he even had time for the stroke.

I remember leaving the church after his memorial and saying to my husband, "We've got to up our game." It seemed like I'd done so little with my life in comparison with my brother. He was a real inspiration and I hope I can manage half of what he accomplished in my senior years.

Patty Lent

Patty Lent was mayor of Bremerton, Washington for eight years, working hard to put the city on the map. Before becoming mayor, she served as county commissioner. When the previous mayor retired, she knew she could make a difference. So, at the age of sixty-four, she ran for and was elected mayor.

"I'm a doer," Patty told me, "and I do have energy." After watching her in action, I must say that is an understatement. Between meetings, phone calls, conferences, ribbon cutting ceremonies, and attending events, a mayor's days and nights are full. It used to exhaust me watching her in action.

"As long as I have energy, good health, enthusiasm and passion, nothing can stop me from accomplishing my goals," she said. I was sad our mayor didn't win her bid for a third term, but I suspect she's already making plans for new adventures.

Sandy Hamilton

Silver fox, Sandy Hamilton, also known as Santa Colorado, is a prolific songwriter. He not only has his songs available for people across the internet to enjoy on a website called Reverbnation, but, as of this writing, he's also brightening up his corner of Colorado by making holiday appearances at local libraries and family-oriented venues in his Santa regalia. Still going strong at seventy-five, he's recording CDs, and has created a charming collection of Christmas songs for children titled *Sleighride with Santa*. One of the things I so admire about this man is the fact that he's always got a plan for the future – a new song to write, open mikes to host, a CD to record. Sandy will never be bored. He doesn't have time!

Bunny McKnight

This lovely woman is no longer with us, and that is a sad loss for the people in Des Moines, Washington who knew her. We've all heard the adage about blooming where you're planted. Bunny did exactly that, devoting herself to mentoring younger women just starting out in married life. Bunny was probably entering her seventies when I met her. She had a problem with her hip and used a cane. She couldn't see well either, and wore glasses with lenses the size of your foot. She had to use a magnifying glass to read. But Bunny had no problem seeing when people were in trouble and needed encouragement.

We were still settling into our new church when I met Bunny, and we had a new baby ... a baby with severe problems. Heather, our firstborn, was microcephalic and had cerebral palsy. She never got beyond functioning on about the level of a four-month-old. When Heather was first diagnosed I was in shock. I couldn't understand how this had happened to us and why God wouldn't heal our baby girl. As time went on I found it increasingly hard to get through a morning church service. Once the singing began I found myself in the women's bathroom, crying, trying to get a grip.

One day, after church, Bunny approached me. "I think the Lord wants me to meet with you," she informed me.

Looking back, I think so, too. At the time I was desperate for answers and I gladly took her up on her offer. I found myself at

Bunny's house on a weekly basis, venting my hurt, my frustration and my anger. I could say anything to Bunny and it never shocked her. She was a world class listener.

She didn't merely listen, though. She also assigned me sections of Scripture to read and instructed me to journal my thoughts. I did. And somehow, in all of this, I began to heal.

Looking back on that time, I realize that we never once talked about Bunny, about her hurts and frustrations. She never complained. She was simply always there.

And not only for me. Bunny took several young women under her wing. I remember fondly enjoying lunches at Bunny's with these other women, and I still make her carrot-tuna salad forty years later. Bunny had her share of health challenges, of griefs and sorrows, but they never stopped her from reaching out to others, being a listening ear and an encouragement. It wasn't a high visibility ministry. She wasn't running a huge non-profit. But she was impacting lives all the same.

Tom Nordlie

Our friend Tom Nordlie is opting to work rather than retire and runs his own business. Mr. Nordlie, as we affectionately call him, and his lovely wife Kathy have been successful, but that success hasn't been luck. It's the fruit of much hard work.

It's not business success, however, that makes this man such a stand-out senior. It's the other things he's doing with his life. He is the vision behind a nature preserve in the town of Poulsbo, Washington, called Fish Park, having been on the steering committee from the park's beginning (as of this writing seventeen years ago). He's devoted countless hours to securing funds, clearing land, and developing trails, giving locals and visitors alike a lovely place to enjoy nature. In 2018 Mr. Nordlie was awarded the well-deserved Governor's Volunteer Service Award in the environment category.

When he's not working on or improving Fish Park, Tom and his wife Kathy are opening their home to friends and neighbors. Tom went to cooking school and is a gourmet chef and eating at their house is a guarantee of a five-star meal. Every fall he hosts a huge fall party, gathering us all to make apple cider. (The Nordlies provides both the apples and the apple press.) We find ourselves out in the crisp air surrounded by boxes and boxes of apples, putting them through the cider press he invested in specifically for this event. Kathy hangs lanterns from the fruit trees and sets up picnic tables a´ la Martha Stewart, with charming checked tablecloths and candles. Everyone brings a side dish to go with the main course, which can be anything from grilled salmon to cioppino. After the work is done, friends gather around the fire pit to visit and recover from their labors. And, of course, he and Kathy insist on us all taking home several bottles of apple cider.

Mr. Nordlie doesn't consider himself a mover and a shaker. As for his elaborate yearly party, that's no big deal. It's just him and his wife having fun with friends. Of course, we all tell them how much we love this event, but sometimes I don't think they get what a cool deal it really is. It's simply business as usual for them.

Ursula Rudorf

Ursula started a café for children in need in her east German town of Weida. Supported by donations, the café not only helps children, but volunteers also reach out to assist the parents when needed, helping them with monthly financial difficulties and fixing broken appliances.

"As long as you're alive you can be useful," she told me when I interviewed her. Ursula has since turned the managing of the café over to her daughter, but she is still being useful, hosting neighborhood gatherings in her home. Last I talked with Ursula, at nearly seventy, she was hoping to become an au pair in Ireland so she could enjoy working with children again and see more of the world.

Bishop Larry Robertson

In addition to pastoring Emmanuel Apostolic Church, Bishop Robertson is a mover and shaker in the town of Bremerton, Washington. At the time of this writing Larry is sixty-six and still going strong. Currently, he's celebrating the completion of a project for which he's had a heart for many years: The Marvin Williams Center, an eight-million-dollar recreation center, designed to provide everything for the community from job training and nutrition education to a place for teens to play after school.

"The vision of the center came when I was in my fifties," says Bishop Robertson. "I was asked by the school district during a long campaign to go around and talk to some of the families. When I saw the devastation in so many families I realized there was a need. I saw poverty, a lack of furniture. Little kids didn't have shoes." He sees the center as a way to centralize resources. "These kids don't have a place around here to go."

They do now, thanks to Bishop Robertson, who has received numerous awards, including a citizenship award from the state of Washington's Secretary of State and a community service award from the Kitsap Community Foundation. Ever since he first had this vision for something that could help the community, he's worked tirelessly to make it happen. The church broke ground for the center in July of 2016, with an impressive collection of dignitaries and politicians present and it is now an impressive building at the center of the city and already being put to good use.

The man is still tireless. "I didn't realize I was getting older," he told me. And he has no plans to retire. "The people who should have been talking to me about retiring weren't thinking about that either."

I asked him what he saw as the role of older people in the church and the community. He said, "The Bible says we call the young because they're strong and the old because they know the way. We need the older people to provide wisdom, encouragement, and direction."

His advice to those who have not joined the mover and shakers club? "Find your passion quickly. You're retiring from work, you're not retiring from your calling."

Laura Knieb

Retirement can give us the opportunity to follow our passion. Laura Knieb, owner of F.R.O.G. Soap, which is not far from Bishop Robertson's church, has found her passion: soap-making. She was fifty-six when she started her business and now, at sixty-two, is going strong and proving that it is easy to be green. She reclaims and uses between three and four hundred pounds of oil a month. Her business has won the prestigious NUCOR Steel Recycler of the Year Award for Washington State. Laura also serves on the Kitsap Solid Waste Advisory Committee as an alternate commercial representative.

And, as if that isn't enough to keep her busy, Laura also served on the board of the Downtown Bremerton Association and made sure downtown Bremerton's Ladies Night Out happens every year. She has recently pared back on some of her community service to keep up with the demands of a growing and increasingly more successful business.

Irene Lennard

Irene says, "I have never been bothered by age. I think it's because I'm more concerned about good health."

She's obviously doing something right because at the time of this writing she's ninety-four and still going strong. She says her mother lived to be ninety-eight and was still enjoying life right up until the day she died. Irene's sister was ninety-nine when she died. "It's left to me to get the letter from Buckingham Palace," says Irene, a transplanted Brit. She's determined to make it to one-hundred and get that congratulatory letter from the Queen Mum. At the rate she's going, I think she will.

Irene is a widow. Although she has no children, she has plenty of friends who are more than happy to give her rides to the local senior center where she does line dancing two days a week. Not content to just go to class, she also opens her home one day a week, holding her own line dancing get-togethers in her basement. Club membership and walks, working in her garden and keeping house all keep her busy and contributing to her community.

Shirley McKnight

"I really resent the societal emphasis on youth," says retired school secretary Shirley McKnight. "And I really respect women who are not doing plastic surgery and buying into the whole youth culture thing."

Shirley doesn't have time to mourn her lost youth. At eighty-one she's too busy being a vibrant and busy senior. Shirley has flair. She has a cool hairstyle, wears hip glasses and stays busy volunteering in our city of Bremerton, Washington. When she's not traveling, she serves on the downtown Ladies' Night Out committee and also on the board of one of our local museums, where she also volunteers. She loves art and volunteers at the local art gallery as well as for a local community theater. In addition to that she also started a book club because she's passionate about reading. Shirley says her father was big on giving back to the community and that's what inspired her.

Shirley has had two cancers. She was in her late seventies when this started. The first one was colon cancer. Following that she beat back uterine cancer. Before chemo she shaved her head, announcing that "Cancer's not going to tell me what to do."

Her advice for anyone starting that final lap in life? "Get out of your house. There are so many opportunities for volunteerism. Get your focus off yourself and onto giving. Find an area that really interests you – hospitals, fine arts, children – all theaters rely on volunteers. And maintain your positive attitude."

JERRY McDONALD

Jerry certainly got out of his house. Another mover and shaker in our city of Bremerton, Washington Jerry became a city councilman at the age of sixty-nine. When he and his wife moved to Bremerton he saw some things he thought should be changed, so decided to run for office. "I knocked on a lot of doors and got elected by forty-two votes," says Jerry. "You only needed to win by one vote. I had forty-one extras." Jerry found satisfaction in some of the things he proposed for the city being put into effect, and one accomplishment he's proud of having gotten security cameras installed on several downtown streets. Jerry's term as councilman has ended but he's now working in other ways to make our city better. He feels that because he's retired he has more time to spend serving the city.

How about you? Want to see some changes where you live? Jerry will tell you to go for it.

BEV AND ED (No last names needed, they told me.)

At seventy-eight and seventy-five Bev and Ed, a retired English teacher and commodities stock broker, became the proud owners of a charming, old Tudor house in our city that was in great need of tender loving care.

Ed was ready to relax and enjoy retirement, but restoring an old home to its former glory was something his wife had always wanted to do so he went along with her. (Ed gets the Good Husband of the Year Award in my book!)

The house required an investment of both time and money. It had stood empty for three years and vandals had broken in and made off with all the copper wiring (not to mention the fireplace mantel). Bev and Ed hauled away seven thousand pounds of old carpet and got busy refurbishing. The house is now not only charming, but it also houses their new business: an espresso café and tea room. The Tudor Roses Meeting House is fast becoming a popular gathering spot.

I was so impressed when I heard who had taken on the project of restoring this old home, I asked for a chance to interview the couple. Giving an old home a new life and starting a new business – who does that in their seventies? After talking with Bev and Ed, I'm convinced the answer to that would be anyone with vision and energy. These two are inspiring.

I asked them for their secrets to staying vital and vibrant. Bev is convinced that having a project keeps you young. Her advice? It stems from something she heard the science fiction writer Ray Bradbury say years ago when he addressed her high school class. "Do in your life what you did when you were young and you'll always be happy." Bev has always loved old houses. Now she's pursuing her passion and she is, indeed, happy. "People said, 'You're too old.' People thought we were crazy," she told me. "We're not crazy. We're passionate." Ed is a proponent of keeping your mind sharp. He's big on puzzles and reading, and he still follows what's going on in the stock market every day. His advice: "Don't be boring." No one will ever accuse this couple of that. It's hard to be boring when you're active and involved in life.

Laura Sargent

At age eighty-one, Laura biked the Allegheny Passage with her son, going from Pittsburgh to Washington D.C. She biked nine miles a day to train for her adventure. Laura told me she hadn't been on a bike in fifteen years, but this was something she thought she'd like to do. Getting to do it with her son, who was retiring, made the adventure even more special. "I never really had a bucket list," she told me. "But if I did this would be on it." So, Laura decided to go for it. She invested in a bicycle and bike pants, which, she jokes, cost nearly as much as the bike, and got busy peddling. She says that her daily bike rides have made her stronger and helped with her balance. I say, "Go Laura!"

Rosemary Dodson

Rosemary may be in a retirement home, but she hasn't retired from life. She's received the resident volunteer of the year award at McCrite Plaza Senior Living in Topeka, Kansas, and has been president of the Residents Council for several years. Eighty-two-year-old Rosemary has arthritis in her hips and back and is in a wheel chair, but she says it's not a problem getting around at all. "I just wheel where I want to go." She's a member of the Red Hat Society and has read poetry and Bible verses to residents who can no longer read. If I ever end up in a retirement home I want to meet a Rosemary! Her sage advice: "Give a prayer in the morning for God to be with you and live every day to its fullest. Keep busy." Obviously, Rosemary is taking her own good advice.

Joanne Berenston

Joanne is eighty-eight and still going strong. She leads a women's Bible study once a month, golfs once a week, and started a game group for several of the widows in her neighborhood. Her game group grew out of her desire to try something new. "I got myself a Mexican Train game for Christmas," she told me.

I loved hearing that. There was no waiting around to see if Santa brought what she wanted. She just went for it. Then she brought her friends in on the fun. In addition to these activities, she's part of a group of women who call themselves the wine widows, and they meet on a regular basis to enjoy a glass of wine, some snacks, and a good visit.

Sam Moyle

My other big brother is a great example of someone who is still using his skills to help others. He had a successful career as a math teacher and high school football coach, but long after retirement, he's still assisting math students with their assignments. Two generations of teens in our large family have called the "math hotline" many times for help with algebra and geometry. At our most recent family Christmas Eve gathering Sam was taking a break from the fun and games to help a great niece puzzle out some tricky problems.

Adeline Short

My grandmother was the first of three women in my family who had a great impact on my life, and I'm betting you have someone similar in your life as well. She never found fame or fortune. Hers was a simple life, but filled with meaning because she invested it so heavily in others. She was widowed young and left on her own to raise her four children. After that she then spent the rest of her life living with first one, then another of them, helping with their families.

Low and behold, when Grandma was sixty-eight, I was born, and Grandma came to live with us to help my mom with her later-in-life baby. Grandma was my mom's right-hand woman, my parents' live-in babysitter, and my pal and my comfort, especially when there was a thunder storm. How I loved crawling in bed with Grandma! I always felt so safe.

As I look back on her life I'm impressed with how determined she was to remain useful. In her eighties she was still stumping up and down the stairs to our basement with laundry and doing the dishes every night. She was a constant example of selflessness, kindness and grace.

FLORENCE MOYLE

My mother was a gifted artist and an excellent writer, but the closest she ever came to fame was writing a column for a local community newspaper in Seattle. She preferred to focus on being the quintessential mom, the kind you see on old TV shows from the fifties. The memory of coming home from school to the aroma of baking cookies is firmly embedded in my mind. (I've carried on that tradition; the fat from eating my own cookies is now firmly embedded on my hips.) In addition to everything she did for our family, Mom watched over the little old ladies in the neighborhood, making sure they had rides to church, treats at Christmas and flowers on May Day.

Even when she got older, she never stopped doing for others. She was in her mid-sixties when our handicapped daughter was born and she became my number one caregiver. My best friend and I had a singing telegram company at the time, and while I was out serenading people, Mom was watching over our baby girl. In addition to that, she made costumes for our company, designing the sequined gold notes our singers wore on their tuxedos and creating elaborate capes and bonnets for our Dickens carolers, who performed in local restaurants during the holidays. Not only was this a huge help to me it was a fun creative outlet she thoroughly enjoyed.

When she wasn't helping me with all my crazy projects she

was baking cookies and distributing them in nursing homes. By her mid-eighties she couldn't get around as well but that didn't stop her from staying politically active, donating to her favorite causes and writing letters to the newspaper editor on a regular basis. She never held an office but I sometimes think she did more for the community than some elected officials.

MARLISS MOYLE

My sister-in-law, who, because of the age difference between us, became like a second mother to me, has always been an inspiration. On top of raising five children, she took in several foster children over the years and then went on to help raise grandchildren. She and my brother have hosted our huge extended family gatherings every Christmas Eve for as long as I can remember. Once my parents got too old to host Thanksgiving, she took that on as well, and at eighty-one she is still in charge of the meal. Extended family gatherings can range in size from twenty-five to forty-five and sometimes at Thanksgiving she hosts a second large family meal to accommodate those family members who can't make the first meal.

Doing for her family has always been her main mission in life, and she still hasn't lost sight of that mission. These are hurried times and it's not always easy to keep families together, but Marliss does that for all of us. This is not the kind of thing that gets any press, but it's so vital. Grown-ups and kids alike need a place where they can find encouragement, heal their wounds, and get ready to go back out into a challenge-filled and stressful world. Her doors are always open for that.

She doesn't stop there. She still volunteers in the lunchroom at a nearby school once a week and babysits her great-great grandchildren.

. . .

I LOOK up to these women in my family, not for their accomplishments, but for their character. Neither my mother nor my grandmother ever retired from doing kind things for others. My sister-in-law

has followed right along in their footsteps. She is the matriarch of our family and a very good one, much beloved!

YOU

Okay, that's enough about everyone else. Let's talk for a moment about you. Hopefully, you're already living your life to the fullest. If, however, you're thinking it could be fuller but are feeling a little stalled out or intimidated, remember, you don't have to be brilliant or talented to have an adventure, and you certainly don't have to be famous to have a purpose. (Although maybe you will go on to become famous.) You don't have to be larger than life or speak to a packed auditorium filled with eager listeners to make an impact. You simply have to be involved in the business of living.

That might mean taking up running or working out with weights. It might mean trying out for a national talent show. Or entering a writing contest. Or taking dance lessons and entering some ballroom competitions.

As you can see by many of the stories I've shared, simply being yourself and reaching out to others can make a big difference. For most of us, influence and inspiration are contained in a small circle.

Don't undervalue your contributions to the world, even if you might think they're small. Little things can make a big difference in the lives of others. Take for example my brother, the king of the math hotline, sends me a card every Valentine's Day. It's only a card but it means a lot. It makes me feel special and I look forward to getting it every year. How much effort does that take him? Obviously, not a lot, but it reminds me that he loves me and opening that card makes my day. So, is it a big thing? No. Is it worth the small amount of time he invests in that sweet gesture? Oh, yes!

That brings us back to you. Is there someone in your family or neighborhood would be encouraged by a small gesture of kindness? You might be the one who's meant to give it.

It's never too late to be useful or do something to make someone smile. There's always something we can do to feel good about ourselves and give our lives meaning. Maybe next election you can stand on a street corner with your favorite candidate, holding a sign and waving at passing cars. Or maybe you can contribute to that campaign. (Or how about running for office yourself?) Maybe you can be instrumental in organizing a neighborhood crime watch or make phone calls to raise money for your favorite charity.

There's also the time-honored tradition of helping with grandkids, which can be a win-win for everyone. Can you take the grandkids for a weekend to give their parents some time to themselves? Can you help with driving kids to and from extracurricular activities? Or, if you're not driving anymore, can you host a granddaughter one afternoon a week for a baking session or some games? The beauty of grandparenting is that grandparents often have time for those little extras, like playing a game together, that working parents don't have. And kids love the extra attention. Helping Grandpa build a birdhouse or playing canasta with Grandma not only gives a child pleasure but it also makes a memory.

If you don't have grandchildren living nearby I'm betting you could find one or two in your neighborhood or at your local church to adopt.

If the kid thing isn't your forte how about picking up the phone and giving someone a call? You might make that person's day. Send an old friend a card to say hi. Or an email. Remember, small gestures can have a big impact.

Even if you're too tired to make a phone call or write a letter, you can still pray for your loved ones, offer a smile for your care-giver or helper or be a listening ear for a relative or friend who's having trouble. Never let anyone make you think that you no longer have value or a place on this earth.

We're all movers and shakers... even if we don't move far and can't shake much.

3. BIBLE STORIES FOR SENIORS

"The righteous will still bear fruit in old age, they will still stay fresh and green."

-Psalm 92:14, the Bible, NIV version

If your parents took you to Sunday School at your neighborhood church when you were a child you might remember these stories about some of the Bible's older heroes and heroines that I'm about to share. If you never did church and are wondering why you should bother now, or even if you know these ancient stories well, I hope you'll indulge me. Now that we ourselves are older I think looking at them can inspire us.

One reason I love these stories is because they are a reminder that, in the eternal scheme of things, no one is too old to find purpose in life. You're never all washed up as long as the cosmic washing machine is still going. In fact, God often tapped people who had a lot of years under their belt.

Take Noah. Noah was five hundred years old when God put him in the boat-building business. Granted, humanity had a much longer life span in those early days of history, but still, at the age of five hundred the man was hardly in the first bloom of youth.

God wasn't interested in Noah's age. He was interested in the man's heart. The people He had created had turned against Him, choosing depravity over righteousness. Finally fed up with His creation, the almighty God said, "Enough. I'm wiping them out and starting over."

Except Noah and his family made the cut, so to speak. Noah, a righteous man, would be spared. Not only spared, but commissioned to build the ship that would house him and his family during the great flood. So, at five hundred years old he began the biggest adventure of his life. Obviously, God found him up to the task.

And what a huge task it was! The ship was to be three hundred cubits long by fifty cubits wide by thirty cubits high.[1] Putting that in terms we moderns can understand, the thing was about five hundred feet long (the length of almost one and a half football fields) with its roof more than fifty feet from the ground. It would have had the same storage capacity as about four hundred and fifty standard semi-trailers. Needless to say, building this was a full-time job! (If you're ever in Williamstown, Kentucky, you can visit a life size model of it.)

By the way, over the years many people have claimed to have found the ark while some insist the story is allegorical. Whether true or allegorical, it is inspiring, and a reminder that one man with a vision can accomplish a lot.

Noah wasn't the only man who had his big adventure in his seasoned years. Think of Abram, father of the Jewish nation, called to leave his homeland and set out for a land ... someplace. Leave the family, leave the kids and grandkids. *Oh, that's right, you don't have any kids or grandkids. But not to worry. You will. In fact, you're going to end up with so many descendants nobody will even be able to count them.*

It took God saying this a couple of times to Abram for it to sink in.

As for his wife Sarai, when she heard the prediction of all their future descendants, she laughed. I probably would have laughed, too. Surely the idea of giving birth at the age of ninety-nine had to sound preposterous.[2] *Yeah, right, God. Tell me another joke.* Menopause was a distant memory. How on earth would she wind up pregnant? No artificial insemination back then. No fertility drugs. Miraculously, God made good on his promise and Abram and Sarai became Abraham and Sarah when she gave birth to a bouncing baby boy, making her husband a father at the age of a hundred.[3]

I sometimes think of Abraham and Sarah, raising a child at such an advanced age, and shudder. Child rearing is an exhausting job, which is why most of us take it on when we're young. But these two are proof that, if God is in it, no job is too hard at any age. Faith and obedience were the keys to their success.

If you're being asked to raise a grandchild or help with child-care, consider the fact that you, like Abraham and Sarah, are being called to embark on an adventure that will possibly affect coming generations. Don't panic. Just as He enabled Abraham and Sarah, God will enable you. Your input may change the life direction of a child and even of that child's children.

We don't talk about Caleb much but I find him very inspiring. When the young nation of Israel stood on the verge of taking their promised land, Caleb was one of the men who'd spied out the land years earlier and came back with a good report. Most of the men who'd been sent ahead to check out the new digs had returned with fearful predictions. "The people in that land are too big and scary for us. We can't do this." Caleb, along with Joshua, said, "Yes, we can. Let's go. Let's take the land God promised us."

The people didn't listen to Caleb and Joshua. They wimped out and a whole generation died before they got a second chance at coming into their inheritance. The only two left from that time were Caleb and Joshua. Joshua led the people into the land. Caleb, too, was ready to roll. In Joshua 14:10 he says to Joshua the commander, "So here I am today, eighty-five years old. I am still as strong as I was then."[4]

This man had confidence and he was ready to claim God's promise for his life. I would be willing to bet he had family members saying, "Dad, you're way too old for this." But he didn't listen, and in the end he saw his dream of life in the new land come true.

What new land lies ahead of you? Be a Caleb and say, "Bring it on. I can do it!"

Moses was a man who had it all. Raised in Pharaoh's palace, educated, given wealth and position, he blew it when, in a rash moment, he killed an Egyptian slave master. He fled for his life and wound up living in obscurity for years. There had to have been times when he remembered the high position he once enjoyed and how much promise he had and bemoaned the choices he'd made as a young man. He had to have wished he could go back in time and undo that horrible deed. He had to wonder what he was doing out in the desert by himself, so far from his people. Perhaps he'd given up on the idea of ever accomplishing anything.

As with Noah and Abraham, God waited until youth was far behind Moses to tap him on the shoulder. At a time in life when he should have been sitting outside his tent letting the younger men chase around after the sheep, a time when he might have figured he was on the downhill side of life, he wound up leading the young nation of Israel out of slavery.

He not only got them out of Egypt, he also became the mediator between God and His people. It was Moses who wrote down God's commands for Israel. It was Moses who led them to the land given to Abraham generations before, the Promised Land.[5]

One thing I really like about Moses's story is the fact that he not only blew it when he was younger but he spent most of his adult life in obscurity. And yet, look what he went on to accomplish. What might be waiting around the corner for us?

Even if you're not called to lead a nation, you may be called to lead a church. Or a study group. Or tutor. Perhaps your local Park and Recreation department needs your skills.

By this time in life we all have the qualifications to lead and to teach. We have the wisdom and knowledge that can only be gained from experience. Because of that we have much to offer. Think how many charitable organizations are looking for people to be mentors and leaders. Might you be one?

Like Naomi, another memorable Bible character, you may wind up being in a position to give valuable advice to the younger generation.

Naomi is one of my favorite characters in the Bible. You can find her story in the book of Ruth. To sum it up, famine came to Israel and she and her husband and sons left the country to settle in the land of Moab, becoming strangers in a strange land. Her sons married Moabite women and it looked like Naomi was there to stay. Until her husband died and then her sons. After that, with no hope and no future, she decided it was time to return home to her roots and her people.

One daughter-in-law remained behind, but the other, Ruth, came with her, sacrificing the opportunity to find a nice Moabite man and start a family. With no husband, no sons, and no grandchildren, it was a sad homecoming for Naomi. In fact, she was so discouraged she actually changed her name to Mara, which meant bitter, and which she felt was a fair reacton to how God had dealt with her.

Naomi's story wasn't over though. God gave her a new purpose. Suddenly, she was confidante and romantic advisor to the young Ruth. Thanks to Naomi's matchmaking, Ruth found Mr. Right. He turned out to be a man named Boaz, and Ruth and Boaz became the great, great grandparents of King David, Israel's most famous king, and part of the lineage of Christ Himself.

As for Naomi, she got a grandchild out of the deal and found herself with a family again. All this from taking her eyes off her own misery and looking out for the younger generation. In spite of her misery, Naomi found purpose in her life.

Here's another older woman who gets mention in the Bible. Her name was Anna and she makes her appearance in the second chapter of the gospel of Luke where we see her at the temple when Mary and Joseph arrive to dedicate the baby Jesus. According to the account she was very old and a prophetess. Anna never left the temple. She was always there, worshipping God, and we're told that, along with a man named Simeon she prophesied great things for the child Jesus. Anna is a good example of someone being at the right place at the right time and stepping forward to play her own small part in a very big history.

Sometimes we can feel purposeless simply because we've failed to open our eyes and see where we're needed next. Naomi's sage advice gave Ruth a new beginning. Perhaps you know someone who might need your counsel and support. Maybe there's a family in your neighborhood in need of a surrogate grandma to bake them cookies or a grandpa to teach the kids how to make a birdhouse.

As long as we're here we still have purpose. However, I'll be the first to admit that faced with health challenges or hardships it can be difficult to see that purpose.

I remember at one point when I was undergoing chemotherapy after being diagnosed with uterine cancer, walking down the street with my husband in the beach town where we had our vacation condo. I'd been dreaming of upgrading to a house where we'd have more room for family and friends. We walked past a piece of land for sale and I thought, *Why bother? I'm probably not going to live.* It was a low point.

I knew I was well again when, one day, several months later, I was looking at a new property and imagining our family all there together enjoying it. Yes, someday I'll be gone and my final real estate will be somewhere in heaven. Meanwhile though, I'm still here, and I believe God expects me to live the life He gave me to the fullest. We recently bought a lot and our family dream home is now complete. I do my best to fill it with family and friends every weekend.

Another thing that came out of that hard time was a memoir about my battle with cancer which, I hope, has encouraged readers who are going through difficult times. When I was first diagnosed, I certainly didn't expect to get anything good out of that experience. But I did.

If you're in the middle of trying times, let me encourage you not to give up hope. You might be going through your own wilderness experience right now, thinking you're of no use to anyone. But God could still have plans for you. Someone in your life might still need your encouragement and advice. Like Moses, you may be in training for the biggest challenge of your life. We make missteps, low points come. But often, during those low points and what seem to be stagnant times we are learning and being prepared for something new. Keep your eyes open and follow Caleb's example. Don't let anyone tell you you're too old.

And now, let me introduce you to one final ancient named Enoch. Enoch is on record as being a godly man. "Enoch walked with God; then he was no more, because God took him away."[6] As in disappeared. One day he was there and the next he wasn't. No lingering illness, no suffering. Just gone and on to the next life. This after three hundred sixty five years of living. (And to think we're impressed when people these days make it to one hundred!) That part of Enoch's story is interesting but what jumps out at me is who followed after him. His descendants were Methuselah (the man who, at seven hundred eighty-two, holds the record for being the longest living human in history), followed by Lamech and then, wait for it... Noah the ark builder.

We don't see any specific accomplishments listed under the name of Enoch, although the fact that he was simply "taken away" and got to dodge death completely is a pretty cool claim to fame. What I want to point out here is the heritage that Enoch left behind him: descendants who had their act together. The family tree he so carefully watered with his good life produced a hero of the Bible.

You may be thinking, I haven't done anything spectacular with my life. But have you raised children who grew up to become responsible adults? Have you encouraged a member of the next generation to get an education? Have you contributed to a charity that helps the underprivileged? Sometimes, although we don't think we're doing anything, we're sowing seeds of greatness in those who will follow us, setting an example for the next generation or paving the way for someone younger to go out and achieve great things. Don't undervalue those conversations, gifts and small acts of charity. They can be seeds that grow into mighty oaks.

Perhaps you're wishing you'd done more with your life, given more. The Bible is full of stories of people who turned their lives around. So take heart and get turning!

These stories, like our own stories, are all different – different people, different circumstances – but they all demonstrate that each one of us has a place in the grand picture of life. Every dot and brush of color, no matter its size, is important. All lives matter!

1. The measurements for the ark can be found in Genesis 6:15.
2. See Genesis 17:17.
3. See Genesis 21:5.
4. Scripture quoted here is from the NIV Bible, Copyright 1984.
5. Moses's story can be found in the Book of Exodus.
6. Genesis 5:24, NIV Bible translation, Copyright 1984.

4. OLDER, WISER, AND WILLING TO WORK

"You are never too old to set a new goal or dream a new dream."
- C.S. Lewis

I DON'T THINK everyone in our current culture got the memo that senior citizens still have value. Age discrimination is a very real thing. Career setbacks can be frustrating. When they come later in life, they can be downright discouraging.

I've seen this to be the case when someone gets laid off toward the end of his or her career. What is the older person's version of the infamous glass ceiling? The gray ceiling? The cracked ceiling? Whatever it is, there does seem to be a point when Corporate America says, "Say there, Hal, isn't it time for you to retire?" Maybe your company was subtle and called the sudden end of your job a lay-off or a restructuring.

I realize not every company operates this way, but many do. Just ask my friend Don. A talented I.T. guy, he found himself suddenly on the outside of the office, looking in long before he qualified for Social Security. The same thing happened to another good friend. He hadn't even hit sixty yet and was the third top salesmen at his company, but that didn't stop the company from letting him go. Whatever happened to a salesman being worth his weight in gold?

One of the hardest things to get past is that feeling of rejection when things go sour. The questions can circle like buzzards. Why did this happen? If my company didn't want me anymore who else will? What am I worth? Am I all washed up? What's the point of trying? This, of course, can hit at any age but I think it gets harder to deal with as we get older because, once more, we see that youth-is- everything attitude come into play.

It's understandable to feel rejected and unappreciated when this happens, and yes, even a little bitter, especially if you've given years to a company. And then there's the fear factor, which brings more questions, scary ones. What now? Am I all washed up? What am I worth? What if I can't get another job? What will I do if my golden parachute rips and I wind up not having enough money to live on?

Fond farewells and early retirement happen. So, what's a person to do?

I can tell you one thing, giving up is not an option. My friend Don decided to become a writer and he's enjoying great success writing and publishing novels. My other friend went on to make good use of his musical talent and is giving voice lessons. He has both knowledge and performance experience to share and now has control over his own life and career path. In addition to teaching he's arranging music and has written his first novel.

We all need purpose and some sort of work to do. I recently talked with an eighty-two-year-old man who is still running his company and has no intention of retiring. "You retire, you die," he told me. Obviously, he's in no hurry to do either.

But let's circle back to the pesky question of what to do if you've been forced into early retirement? Let me pass on some sage counsel kindly shared with me for this book by Steven Fulmer, speaker, trainer, life coach and author of the book *Leader-*

ship Just Got Personal.[1] When we chatted, his first words of advice were, "Don't panic. It's distinctly likely you are raging with one or more emotions: anger, frustration, sadness, disappointment, joy, worry, excitement, fear, anxiety, numbness, doubt – to name just a few. Whatever it is, start with genuine permission to feel it all, deep into your soul. Let it serve you, inform you, empower you and relax you, because when you resist it, whatever the emotion is, it will cause you to tense up, question everything, judge yourself unfairly, judge the person who 'retired' you even more unfairly or worse, it will give away your power, create weakness, cloud your vision and fog your mind." After that, Steven advises you to ask yourself in what ways this early retirement might be a good thing. "What negative parts of the job do you now get to let go of? How is this a blessing in disguise?"

You may be thinking, *Yeah right. This is not a blessing. It's a curse.* Let me take a moment to share a personal story from several years back in my writing career. My agent dumped me. Not because she was mean but because she needed to earn a living and at the time we weren't having any luck selling any of my book ideas. At the time publishing was in the middle of what was dubbed the midlist crisis. (There's always a crisis in publishing, but that's another story.) There was space on bookstore shelves for exciting new books by authors who'd just been discovered and space for the big names, but those of us dangling halfway up the ladder were in trouble. I was definitely in trouble, even before my agent waved good-bye. My last book hadn't done as well as hoped and my editor was conveniently never in when I called to talk to her. In short, no one wanted me. I was devastated, mortified, discouraged and depressed.

What now? I thought miserably. What would become of me? Who was I if I wasn't a writer?

Happily, after a period of hiding from my writing friends and licking my wounds, I came to realize I was many things. I was a wife, a mom, a friend, a child of God. I had great people in my life, including a supportive husband, and I wasn't starving on the streets.

I reminded myself that I was still creative. Surely there was something in me worth sharing. I just had to dig around and find it.

I slowly began to reinvent myself, exploring new ideas. It took a good year to figure out who I was, but finally, with some new projects in hand I put myself back out on the market and began the hunt for a new literary agent. Lo and behold, after the agent of my dreams said, "Thanks but no thanks," a writing pal passed on a name. This agent was young and hungry. Maybe she'd be a good fit.

She turned out to be more than just a good fit. She turned out to be the best thing that ever happened to me (in my career, at least). Our start was slow, but she stuck with me. We finally made a great sale and that got me back in the door of the publishing world. Many books and two made-for-TV movies later we're still working together and good friends.

My writer girl version of a lay-off freed me to explore new ideas and become a whole new person. But before that could happen I had to come to grips with my situation. I had to quit feeling sorry for myself and find answers for the all-important question, "What now?" I had to cast a new vision and turn myself in a new direction. I had to believe that I could still get out there and do something. I had to tell myself that I wasn't a failure. I'd only hit a roadblock and needed to find a new route to take me where I wanted to go.

I look back at that miserable interlude in my career and smile and shake my head. I was so sure my life was over when in reality it was about to take a big turn for the better. Maybe yours is too!

Steven says, "Regardless of whether early retirement is a good ending or a sad ending, it is an ending nonetheless. Let it end." Once you let go you are then free to turn your life in a new direction. According to Steven, it doesn't matter where you are in your career. It matters *who* you are. So, with that in mind, if you're wanting to start a new direction, a new adventure, a new job, here is Steven's advice for how to start in a new direction and find a new home for your skills:

"Start by naming every single organization that looks like they are doing the work you want to be doing in the world. Then find somebody in that organization you can reach and ask for an informal interview. Ask for fifteen minutes of that person's time to ask about the company." Steven says that won't work every time but it will work better than fifty percent of the time "because people like to help people."

"Once you get an interview be prepared with questions about the company's culture and why they do what they do the way they do it," he says. "Ask about their five-year plan and what kind of people thrive there and what kind don't. When you're reaching the fifteen minute mark, name it and thank the person for his or her time. The person will appreciate that and might even ask how else he or she can help you, a possible open door."

In your resume, Steven advises, "Begin to formulate your story by identifying how your experiences could help solve the company's problems and compliment their culture." He also says, "It doesn't always matter where you got the experience. What matters is that you have it. But if you rely on them seeing the connection between your past and their future, well, they don't have that kind of time. But you do. So help them make the connection."

I'd like to add another piece of advice to that. If it's been a while since you've done a resume, enlist the help of a young professional with creativity and good copywriting skills to help you. This may feel like conflicting advice. After all, we're fabulous the way we are with our years of experience and wisdom, right? Right. But it's also good to show that we are not dinosaurs, that we can adapt to changes in the business world, and in spite of the years under our belt our thinking is fresh and our talents relevant. Also, let me point out that every professional writer has an editor to look over his or her work and make sure it's ready for Prime Time. Your resume is an equally important work so don't be afraid to get help with producing it. A creative and impressive resume can open doors.

If you don't know anyone who can help you, check with your local library. Libraries often offer classes in resume writing. Even if your local library doesn't offer this sort of class, your librarian can probably point you to some helpful resources. Librarians know things! You can also find a plethora of information on how to write resumes on the internet.

Of course, these days it's all about searching and being found on the internet, so you'll want to make sure you're visible on various networking and job boards. Look for sites that list openings exclusively in your area of interest and expertise. And be sure to sign up for RFF feeds (automatic electronic information sharing system) that allow you to receive content in an easy to read format.

Here are some other to-dos that I found poking around online:

When an ad lists a hiring contact, research the person's background to see if you might have a special connection. (Perhaps you have the same alma mater?)

If an employer's career page invites visitors to fill out a candidate profile, do it. If a position opens up that matches your profile, you'll receive an email notifying you.

Use filters if a job board offers this tool. That way you can refine your search and not waste time wading through other job offers that have nothing to do with what you want. Filters are usually located on the left side of the results page.

Most of us are familiar with LinkedIn and Monster, but there are other boards as well (at least at the time of this writing) such as SimplyHired, Us.jobs, and TheLadders, a board that focuses on job openings for upper-level executives.

If you need to retrain in order to launch yourself in a new direction, check with your local community college to see what courses they offer. Chances are you'll find continuing education opportunities in all kinds of fields, ranging from medical billing to trade skills to flagger training.

Perhaps you've had it with working for other people or no one seems interested in hiring you. Consider starting your own business. Let your expertise work for you and offer your services as a consultant. Rent space in your town's downtown area or local mall for the holidays and try a pop-up store. If bonbons and cookies are your thing, get the necessary food license and see if you can rent or borrow a commercial kitchen to create goodies to sell at craft fairs. Your local church or service club might have a kitchen you can use. Become an Uber or Lyft driver, start a daycare business, hire yourself out as a gardening or computer tech expert. Sell kitchen tools at home parties. Write a novel or become a publicist and help other writers promote their books. (If my writing career crashes that's my next choice!) Become a party planner. Get into real estate. Work on cars.

There truly are so many possibilities. But if you're drawing a blank, sit down with a couple of friends, ask them what they think you're good at, and brainstorm ideas for how to turn that into an occupation. While you're brainstorming, here are some other questions you can ask yourself to see if self-employment will work for you:

Do I have access to the money I need to start my business?

Most businesses require a certain amount of money to breathe life into them. Do you have the necessary start-up funds so you can do what you want to do? Also, do you have money to live on while you're doing what you want to do? (Money in savings or a spouse still working?)

Of course, there are loans available for small business startups from such sources as the Small Business Administration, but my feeling is that at this point in life the less debt we shoulder the better. Still, you can find ways to get creative, using options such as GoFundMe.

How brave am I?

If you're going to get out there and start a new business you have to be brave enough to make contacts, network, close deals. You have to be brave enough that the thought of possible failure doesn't terrify you. Are you thick-skinned enough to be able to take no for an answer?

Am I a self-starter?

You are the boss and the employee of your company. And both of you have to show up every day, all day. If you're an ambitious self-starter this won't be a problem for you.

Do I manage my time well?

If you answered yes to the previous question, you'll probably answer yes to this one as well. And that's a good thing. You know the old adage, time is money. And when you're working for yourself, you can't afford to waste it. If you were easily distracted working for someone you might be just as easily distracted when working for yourself. By the way, having had my own business I can assure you that it's not so much you owning the business, but the business owning you, especially when you're first starting up.

Am I in good enough health to take on the responsibility of a new venture?

It's easy to get carried away with the dream of finally getting to__________ (you fill in the blank), but you make sure you have the stamina to do it.

Do I have people in my corner?

Have you got family members or friends who will cheer you on? Are any of them willing to help you with writing a business plan, filling orders, bookkeeping, making sales calls? Remember, when starting a business you want to start small and carefully. If you have a spouse or sibling who will work for free (or an occasional dinner out), that's a good thing.

. . .

THOSE OF US who have always worked might be ready for a change. If you don't need the money but want to fill your time in a satisfying way, find a worthwhile organization and volunteer your skills. Volunteers are a rare breed and wherever you decide to plug in you are bound to be appreciated. Volunteerism is one of the best ways to find purpose and meaning in your life, and whereas the corporate world may think it doesn't need you anymore, the world of charities and non-profits will most likely welcome you with open arms.

I like my dancing pal Alan's philosophy of life. He says he's on the ninety-year plan. According to Alan, the first thirty years of life are for living. The second thirty are for making your learning count (as in work/career). The third thirty years are for giving back. Maybe you've reached the point in life where you can enjoy giving back.

Sandy Harley, the Executive Director of the food bank in Ocean Shores, Washington, is enjoying giving back. She says she's "proud to be a seasoned and wise seventy-one." She is a good example of how retirement can free you to go on to do even more important things than what you were doing to earn a paycheck.

She and her husband Bob fell in love with Ocean Shores and its people and decided to retire there. They became involved in the community and she started volunteering for an event that raises money for our local animal shelters and contributes to the food bank so they can buy pet food to distribute to pet owners who are experiencing hard times. One thing led to another and soon Sandy was also volunteering for the food bank. Her experience in the corporate world made her a natural choice when a new Executive Director was needed. Last time we chatted about the food bank Sandy told me that to date it had distributed 976 tons of food and served 4,846 households. That's a lot of needs being met. "Frankly," she says, "my life has become even more enriched since my involvement with the food bank."

Sandy encourages every senior to stay active, maintain old friendships, and develop new ones. "Follow your heart and go where God is leading you," she advises.

When I asked her what she thought older citizens can contribute to the world she said, "I think our biggest gift that we can share is our life experiences. I would hope that we can set an example to the younger generation to show love and compassion toward each other. I would also hope that, as older citizens, we share the joy of serving and helping others. I think it's especially important to instill that in children today. They need good role models." Well said, Sandy! And well done.

Perhaps you could be teaching a younger generation how to knit, how to write, how to paint. Maybe it's time you started a blog or wrote a column for your local paper. Or, like my buddy Elizabeth, a former English professor, you may be able to help budding writers by editing their work. Elizabeth isn't exactly getting rich sharing her expertise but she's certainly helping a lot of people achieve their dreams.

Whether it's a church, a service organization, or a non-profit, there is always a need for wiser and experienced heads to guide. There are certain lessons about life and human nature that take time to learn. We have (hopefully) learned those lessons, and we're in a position to advise and help those who are not as far along on their life journey.

Whatever you wind up doing, know that you're not doing it too late. Don't talk yourself out of trying new things because you think you're too old. There are opportunities out there waiting for you and new roads to take. There is still money to be made and there are plenty of organizations that will appreciate your skills. Don't let fear keep you from branching out in a new direction.

And don't rationalize not trying by saying things like, "It probably wouldn't happen anyway." Maybe "it" wouldn't, but you won't know unless you try.

I have been talking about going on the TV show *Dancing with the Stars* ever since that show first came on TV. I talked about it to everyone – to my family, my friends, readers – even my literary agent. I remember the first time I mentioned that particular dream to her. We'd just made a deal for my novel *On Strike for Christmas* to be made into a movie for TV. Needless to say, I was excited. "So, do you think you can get me on *Dancing with the Stars?*" I asked eagerly.

"Sheila," she said gently, "You'll always be a star to me. And no offense, but don't you have to be famous?"

"Well, can't you make me famous?" I replied.

My agent is great, but getting me on TV isn't exactly in her job description. So I kept dreaming and talking and dreaming and talking.

Finally, I hired a publicist and suckered her into helping me make contact with the producer of the show. We made an audition tape and sent it in. And no, no one has called me yet to invite me on the show.

But at least I tried. I threw my hat in the ring and I am now "in the files" which I suspect means, "Don't call us, we'll call you." All right. I can take no for an answer (God just has to shout it at me!) The point of this is that now I can be okay with it if that dream doesn't come true because I did everything in my power to make it happen. If I hadn't gone ahead and tried, I'd still be talking and dreaming and a little frustrated because I wasn't where I wanted to be.

The moral of this little story is get out there and go and do. You never know what might happen. One thing you can be sure of, you have a better chance of something happening than if you do nothing.

My friend Debbie Macomber has been writing for years, and she's still going strong both as a writer and a much in demand public speaker. She once told me you have to have a dream. When you stop dreaming you die.

Actually, we're all going to die no matter how many dreams

we have, but Debbie made a good point. Part of being alive is dreaming – setting goals and making plans. In short, living our lives. Yes, as we get older we may experience some limitations, but that doesn't necessarily mean we're out of the race. You don't have to be the fastest runner to stay on the track.

One of my favorite quotes is from Walt Disney, who said, "If you can dream it you can do it." He certainly proved that when he created Disneyland.

Perhaps you're not in a position to build the next Disneyland, but you might be in a position to build a house or a whole new life. Or maybe help start a new church or a school. Perhaps you'll go to Africa and help build wells. Or volunteer for Habit for Humanity like former president Jimmy Carter. What are you dreaming? Maybe now's the time to make that dream come true.

I love the Bible verse, Philippians 4:13. It reminds me I can do all things thanks to the strength God gives me. If God has a new road for me to travel, I can walk down it with confidence, knowing He'll give me the strength I need.

As long as we're here, we're here for a reason. Find yours and do what you're meant to do. Don't let the end of one adventure stop you from embarking on a new one.

1. Steven Fulmer, *Leadership Just Got Personal*, (Steven Fulmer Inc., 2012).

5. TO YOUR HEALTH

When did you first notice those body aches? The fact that you couldn't run quite as fast or work in the yard quite as long? I think it first hit me in my early sixties.

I still remember one of my friends saying, "Just wait till you turn sixty. Everything starts falling apart."

"Well, it's not going to happen to me," I replied.

Silly me. It did. Uterine cancer struck at sixty-two. Happily, I was able to fight it off, but other smaller irritations stepped in to take its place. Osteopenia thanks to chemo, a trashed rotator cuff, and wear on my knees took their toll, and none of them boded well for my tennis game. I'm still here though, and happy to be, even if I'm not as fit as I was when I was in my thirties.

Perhaps those aches and pains have gotten to you. Maybe you're now fighting the beginnings of some serious disease. Or maybe you're simply feeling tired and frustrated that you feel tired. I hope this chapter will help and encourage you. Yes, we're all going to face health challenges as we age, but there are things we can do to help ourselves stay as fit as possible for as long as possible. And the good news is, there are plenty of books out there to help us, some of which I quote from in this chapter.

Let's start out with some advice from my doctor, Sundance

Rogers, M.D., who, conveniently for me, has switched from being a general practitioner to treating geriatric patients. I asked her to share her advice for those of us who are now seniors. Here's what she had to say:

"Sheila, I think the most important 'secret' to staying healthy is staying active. Every senior I have that is defying their age is active, whether it be with Tai Chi or line dancing, hiking or swimming, it is something. After 50, if you don't use it you definitely lose it. And, once lost at that age it is almost impossible to get back. We know if you lose your ability to balance on one leg, you cannot reteach yourself how to do it. I think staying engaged mentally is also very important. Keeping your mind sharp with reading, card games, book groups, etc., whatever floats your boat, keeps you mentally healthy and if you are going to live forever you want to do it in your right mind!"

This lines up with what physical therapist, Robert Burns, told me: "Find something you love to do and keep doing it."

Let's break down some of this advice, starting with staying active. According to John Medina, developmental molecular biologist and author of the book *Brain Rules For Aging Well*[1] – a book I highly recommend – a number of studies are showing a correlation between exercise and a well-functioning brain.

Do you have a favorite sport or physical activity? Gardening may not get your heartrate up but it will keep you moving, especially if you get up and down to weed or find yourself mowing the lawn or pushing around wheelbarrows of dirt or bark. Instead of hiring someone to rake your leaves come fall, get out and do it yourself.

Writer Colleen Reece, in her eighties at the time, never let a little thing like undergoing chemotherapy for breast cancer stop her from raking her leaves. Our friend Bill just had his eightieth birthday and he's still an avid gardener. He and his wife Sandy moved to a new house in an active retirement community and he was out in their yard, cutting down trees and pulling stumps only last summer. Sandy is staying fit as a dancing queen, enjoying both ballroom and clog dancing.

Speaking of that, maybe dancing is your thing. Or maybe you'd like it to be your thing. It's never too late to sign up for dance classes, even if you've lost your mate. Men, do you want to be the most popular guy on the planet? Learn to dance and then find a night spot or join a fraternal order such as the Elks or Eagles where you can keep your skills sharp. You will find plenty of women happy to help you with that. Ladies, if you're on your own and haven't found a dance buddy, try line dancing. Line dancing clubs are all over the country, and often your local senior center or country music bar will offer line dancing classes. The beauty of dancing is that you are using both your body and your brain as you learn and execute (and remember) new steps. In fact, according to a study by the Albert Einstein College of Medicine, dancing can reduce our risk of dementia more than any other type of physical activity.[2]

Tennis is another sport that gets good ratings, and it's one many of us seniors can manage. I play with a group where the ages range from fifty-something to eighty-something. Most of these players are still moving and hitting great. One of them recently emailed me an article from the *New York Times* purporting that people who play tennis, badminton, or soccer tend to live longer than those who cycle, swim or jog.[3] Who knew?

If tennis is becoming too strenuous you might try pickle ball, a game that originated in the Pacific Northwest but is catching on all over America. It's similar to tennis but the court is smaller so you don't have to run as much or as far. Or table tennis (ping pong). Believe it or not, you can get a pretty good workout at that small table, and you can play year round, even if it snows. Golf is also good, if you're walking the course. Riding around in the little golf cart isn't going to give you much exercise.

The bottom line here is, stay active. Even if sports aren't your thing you can still walk. Take the stairs at your condo instead of the elevator. Go to the gym. Physical therapist Robert Burns tells me that just a few minutes on the elliptical machine is worth twenty on the treadmill.

There are many advantages of hitting the gym, and one of them is that those weight workouts will keep your bones strong. According to Chris Crowley and Henry S. Lodge, M.D., authors of *Younger Next Year*[4], we start to lose bone density after the age of thirty. By the age of sixty we're up to a thirty percent bone loss. To help combat this they advise adequate calcium intake and weight resistance exercise. Current research indicates we need high-impact, weight-bearing exercise to build bone. Since all that high impact jumping around can be hard on the joints, these two authors recommend strength training.

Can you afford to spend three mornings or afternoons at the gym? If you want to keep your bones, can you afford not to? If you can't get to a gym, perhaps an easy workout with light weights might be a possibility.

The good *Younger Next Year* doctors also recommend yoga because it integrates strength and balance (yes that again) training. They suggest you get fit before you start turning yourself into a pretzel though, so you don't injure yourself. Good advice for any new physical activity you pick up. Start slowly.

Maybe you're not quite ready for a yoga class. How can you still work on keeping your balance? Here's a nifty trick. Make like a flamingo and stand on one leg when brushing your teeth. Alternate legs. And stay near the counter so if you start to list to one side you won't fall over. I'm currently doing physical therapy for tendinopathy in my right glut and one of the exercises my physical therapist has me doing is... you guessed it. Alternate standing on one leg. (You can do this while you're standing in front of the mirror brushing your teeth.) If you're big on sports, working on your balance will also help you stay more stable when playing.

Getting in touch with your inner flamingo probably seems

like a little thing, but those little things add up. Parking at the far end of the mall or grocery store parking lot instead of near the entrance gives you some extra steps. If you're still working (and why shouldn't you be if you want to!) getting up from your desk once in a while and walking around is good for your circulation. So is refraining from crossing your legs. Many of us grew up as leg crossers. If you were sitting with my physical therapist right now, he'd point to those crossed legs and say, "Don't do that." Not only is it bad for your circulation, it also puts you out of alignment.

When I was going for physical therapy for my latest sports injury, yet another therapist recommended hitting the swimming pool. Good exercise but less stress on the body. If you're already swimming laps or doing pool exercises, good on ya. If not and you're wanting to move without overstressing your muscles the pool could be the place for you. Many pools have a section that simulates a river and doing the "river walk" will give you a really good workout. So will water aerobics. If that all sounds too strenuous, get in the water and walk back and forth across the pool, forward, backwards and sideways.

You might not be able to afford a gym membership but walking around your neighborhood with a friend won't cost you anything. Also, small hand weights are very affordable, and you can use them while listening to your favorite music or an audio book.

Our bodies were designed to move, but these days many of us aren't moving nearly enough. We have sedentary jobs or hobbies, and probably most of us spend a good deal of time in front of the television or our computers, catching up with friends on Facebook. Of course, the more we sit, the less energy we use and the more fat we store. Pretty soon, before we know it, nothing's fitting, our knees and hips are hurting, and we're riding around the store in a little cart (still sitting, probably buying things that are going to make us heavier and put more stress on our knees and hips).

Did you notice that, when offering her advice, Dr. Rogers didn't mention sitting and watching TV as a way to keep our minds sharp? After a busy day, it's so easy to flop in front of the tube and turn into a turnip. We all have our favorite shows, of course, and I wouldn't want to deprive you of watching yours. But how about building time into your day and your week for both sedentary and physical activities? It's not too late. Remember Laura Sargent, who's becoming a marathon cyclist at eighty-one!

When it comes to physical activity, one final bit of advice that is often only half-jokingly delivered says don't fall down. Well, duh. But, elementary as that may seem, my dear Watson, we all know that a fall can be the beginning of real trouble. Our reflexes and balance aren't what they were when we were twenty and it's easy to tilt toward the floor. One medical expert told me that it's important to remember that we can get thrown off balance and to slow down. Take your time getting up and getting to where you want to go. Quick movements can herald a loss of balance and thus a fall.

In addition to slowing down, here are some other tips. Don't bend over to put on or tie your shoes. Stop and sit down. Don't go crazy on the _______ (you name it: basketball court, tennis court, pickle ball court, dance floor). Over the last few years I've seen plenty of seniors trip on the tennis court and do some serious damage, often while racing for shots they probably should have let go by. And, speaking of racing, don't race for the phone. If you're sitting and watching TV, keep it handy.

My other half recently was putting away some laundry in our dresser while I was out, heard the phone ring, and made a dash to answer it, thinking it might be me. In his haste, he misjudged a turn and ran into a wall, clunking himself in the head. Imagine my surprise coming home to find a note saying, "Be Right Back," followed by my husband returning from the emergency room after having to get stitches. Okay, enough said about that, right?

If you stay mentally as well as physically active you'll really be ahead of the game. Reading, doing any kind of puzzles, picking up a new hobby, learning a new skill or a new game – all of these activities can keep your brain busy and happy.

Get together with a group of friends and play Mexican Train or Bridge. Host a game night and play Charades. Or simply get on your smart phone and play one of the many online games available (Words with Friends, Word Crack, Trivia Crack, Tetris, Plants Vs Zombies, to name a few.) If you're not into the whole technology thing, you can still pop into your local bookstore and pick up a novel or a book of crossword puzzles, Sudoku, and a jigsaw puzzle or two. Or read a mystery and try to figure out in advance who done it. Try and write a mystery. (This, I learned firsthand, is not as easy as it looks.) For that matter, try to write anything – a short story, a poem, a list of your favorite things! Learn a new language (especially good for building brain muscle). Whatever you do, don't just sit and vegetate. Watching TV requires some brain activity, obviously – you have to follow what's going on – but chances are it's not going to get things sparking as much as something that involves more interaction and more brain-hand cooperation. Picking up a new hobby such as wood working, gardening, knitting or crocheting will definitely get both your brain and your hands working. Every time you have to learn new rules or new ways of doing something you pick up brain power. And don't forget those dance classes!

If we're going to keep active, we need to keep fueled. We all know about eating right, but let's refresh our memories on a few no-nos.

Sugar

Yes, we all know about how bad too much added sugar is for us, and if you're a sugar addict like me, this is not a fun topic. But let's address it anyway.

We find sugar in its natural habitat in fruits, vegetables, grains and dairy. And eating whole foods that include it is fine. (I'm sorry to have to say that a whole chocolate cake doesn't count as a whole food.) Added sugar is the problem, and we find that everywhere: soft drinks, fruit drinks, cookies, cake, candy, soups, yogurt, cereals, salad dressings, granola bars, pasta sauces, and ketchup. Sigh.

According to the Harvard University's health website, high amounts of sugar can overload our livers, raise our blood pressure and increase chronic inflammation.[5] Then, of course, we have the problem of added weight gain, which can bring with it diabetes as well as extra wear and tear on our hips and knees.

So, how to get control of this? For me, the answer is to make baking a rare occurrence because if I bake cookies (or pie or cake or... you name it) guess who eats most of it. Yes, little me. These days a cookie is a rare treat. If you love to bake you might want to search for more nutritious recipes that use less sugar and plenty of whole grains and nuts. Or bake up a storm and take your creation to a party to share the fat, er, fun. Better yet, train your palette to appreciate treats that are better for you.

The American Heart Association suggests starting out eating better by cutting the usual amount of sugar you add to things by half and wean down from there. Instead of adding brown sugar to your oatmeal, sweeten it with fruit, and avoid fruit canned in syrup.

As for snacking, get your crunch on with almonds and walnuts, which are good sources of anti-oxidants. Or try some cashews, which are rich in iron, magnesium, zinc, copper, phosphorous and manganese. When your sweet tooth starts begging for a treat give it some dark chocolate. (Yes, sadly, that yummy milk chocolate isn't good for us. If the idea of eating that nasty dark stuff doesn't appeal, let me tell you, try it for a while. Eventually you will come to prefer it. Ha! Never thought I'd hear myself say that.)

. . .

Soft Drinks

An ice-cold cola on a hot day – yum! But if you haven't pared this treat out of your family's life yet you might want to consider it. According to several nutrition websites, studies have linked consuming sugary drinks on a regular basis to increased risk for Type 2 Diabetes, higher risk of heart attack in men, gout (gout!) in women, and obesity. There seems to be some disagreement on this, but most of the material I've read over the years suggests that soda may also pose a threat to our bones and our teeth. Why? It contains phosphate and if we happen to consume more phosphate than calcium we've got trouble. (By the way, if you're wanting to get more calcium in your diet, remember, there are more sources of calcium than milk and cheese. Leafy green vegetables and broccoli will provide you with calcium as well as vitamin K, which is also necessary for good bone health. Almond milk is good also, and works great in smoothies.)

If you're craving a bubbly drink, it would appear your best bet is to drink carbonated water such as seltzer water with fresh fruits or cucumbers added. And, actually, plain old water with sliced cucumber or cubed honeydew melon is great.

Saturated and Trans Fats

I swear, this eating right can take a lot of the fun out of life. But then, so can heart attacks and dying early. According to the American Heart Association (yes them again), saturated fat is bad stuff. We find it in red meats, whole-fat dairy products, and coconut oil. And then there are those trans fats. Stick margarine and the glaze on doughnuts are trans fats. Studies have shown that the more trans fats a person consumes, the faster the cardiovascular system ages. Many packaged foods, such as cookies, crackers and chips (wah) have these trans fats hidden in them. The AHA recommends a diet that gives us only five to six percent of our calories from saturated fats.[6]

Use vegetable oils in recipes that call for butter or margarine. I'll be the first to admit, I'm not there yet. I have definitely given margarine the heave-ho, but I must confess, you'll still find butter in my fridge because I still subscribe to the belief that everything's better with butter, at least when you're baking. (Rarely. Honest.) I do use olive oil and eat my avocados, and I hope you do, also. Avocados are rich in good-for-you fats and are also high in fiber, beta carotene and potassium. And they're rich in vitamin E, which is good for our hearts.

Red Meats

I visited a number of websites to see what the latest consensus was on this, and it seemed to be that we do need to limit our red meat (beef, pork, and lamb) consumption. Over the years, studies have linked its consumption to heart disease, diabetes and cancer. However, new studies are always being done and new studies seem to indicate red meat also provides ten percent of the iron needed to support red blood cell production and supplies and gives us forty percent of vitamins B6 and B3, which help support our nervous and immune systems as well as vitamins A and D. And, of course, it's an excellent source of protein and those amino acids we all need.

But then, so are chicken and fish, and they aren't high in the unsaturated fats like red meat. Fish, in fact, is high in what experts call "good fats," the main one being omega-3. Fish also contains selenium, which is a known cancer fighter.

Here's the bottom line. None of us need to be eating steak, hamburger and pork chops every night. Change it up. Have a meatless night once a week. Enjoy a bean burrito or a fish taco. Or a nice slice of chicken and a salad.

Processed Meats

Meeting with a nutritionist after my battle with uterine cancer, I learned anything that's been salted, cured, fermented or smoked is not good for us. This includes breakfast and lunch favorites such as cold cuts and bacon. Nitrates are not our friends.

My husband and I have cut back on these food items, but honestly, we still want to live a little. So when we do buy sandwich meat or turkey bacon we make sure it's nitrate free. You might want to also.

There are some no-no's. How about some yes-yeses? Like ...

A Good Diet

Rebecca Katz, author of *The Healthy Mind Cookbook*, says, "What we put on the end of our fork definitely affects the brain in a myriad of ways."[7] What are you putting on your fork? If you're putting on lots of dark green leafy vegetables (kale, spinach, Swiss chard) you're increasing your intake of B vitamins, all of which can improve your cognitive function. You're kickstarting the growth of new neurons if you're consuming foods rich in Omega 3's. (Fish, it's what's for dinner.) Add to that foods rich in vitamin E and flavanols (nuts, seeds, broccoli and citrus fruits) and you'll be doing well. Walnuts are especially good for you. (A quick aside here. You may have certain diet restrictions due to medications your doctor has prescribed, so do make sure you can enjoy large amounts of these foods before buying going all out at the grocery store.)

Now, what if you're not eating a well-balanced, healthful, low fat, Mediterranean, you-name-it diet? That brings me to my next recommendation.

Supplements

When it comes to the subject of supplements, people seem to be divided into two camps. We have those who believe eating the right foods will be enough. "Don't get taken in by all those false claims," they say. My eye doctor definitely falls into this category. "You don't have to take any special vitamins," he tells me every time I go in for a check-up.

I nod, and then go out and buy my eye vitamins. You can tell which camp I fall into.

I happen to agree with the experts who say most of us don't eat a well enough balanced diet and our soils are depleted of many necessary vitamins and minerals. So my other half and I supplement our diet with multi-vitamins and minerals. I also take horse chestnut extract for my veins, a collection of goodies to support my adrenals and my turkey tail mushrooms, which are purported to support the immune system and which I've taken ever since winning my battle with uterine cancer. That's just me. You may not want to have an entire cupboard filled with vitamins.

You might, however, want to at least take a good multi-vitamin and some calcium. According to Henry S. Lodge, M.D., our *Younger Next Year* doctor, we should be taking 600 mg of calcium in the morning and another 600 at night. And vitamin D (800 IU). Many vitamins combine these two. I would certainly at least do that. Of course, it's great if you can get your vitamins from all those good foods you're preparing, but the truth is, a lot of us don't spend as much time in the kitchen as we once did. As far as I know, no one ever died from taking a multi-vitamin and some calcium.

I'm not your doctor, so you need to consult your resident expert when deciding what you should be ingesting. Dr. Sheila's only qualifications for doling out advice are a lot of reading, medical shows, and her hypochondria. Do your own research on this subject, talk with your doctor and then make your own informed decisions.

. . .

Aspirin

You've probably heard somewhere that you should be taking a baby aspirin every day. Why? Well, according to Dr. Michael F. Roizen M.D., author of *Real Age: Are you as Young as You Can Be?* taking an aspirin or even half an aspirin a day will keep your arteries free of buildup and helps keep your arteries free from clots by inhibiting an enzyme system called the prostaglandin system (say that fast five times!) that causes platelets to stick together. According to the good doctor, studies on aspirin and aspirin-related drugs have shown a decrease in the incidence of strokes, especially the small ones that are often associated with memory loss. And use of aspirin and other NSAIDs (non-steroidal anti-inflammatory drugs) has been shown to reduce the incidence of Alzheimer's disease, according to the doctor, presumably because it helps keep the arteries in the brain young. Additionally, taking an aspirin a day seems to reduce the incidence of certain kinds of colon cancer. It would appear that the benefits come over time and Dr. Roizen estimates that you need to be taking your aspirin for at least three years to get the full benefit. And the benefits are lost once you stop.[8]

For a long time we were advised to take a baby aspirin (low dose, 81 mg) daily. And this still seems to be the case for those of us who've had a heart episode. If you have stomach issues make sure you buy aspirin that is coated. Even more important, before you run to the drug store and start pulling down bottles, check with your doctor. (Yes, that again.) I personally can't do aspirin every day, partly because it doesn't always make my stomach happy, even the coated variety.

Aspirin and all other NSAID's don't always make other body parts happy, either, such as hemorrhoids. In fact, too many NSAID's can cause ulcers. You may have seen the notice on that ibuprofen bottle warning people over the age of sixty about taking the stuff. This is because NSAIDs have side effects that include upset stomach, heartburn, nausea, constipation, and dizziness. People who are older than 65 are more likely to have serious side effects, like intestinal bleeding or upset stomach. NSAIDs also may cause high blood pressure and have been linked to heart disease. Speaking of, if you are on blood thinners this probably won't be an option for you. (Of course, if you are on blood thinners your doctor or pharmacist has probably already told you this.)

If you have kidney problems or if you are older than sixty-five, talk to your doctor before you start any anti-inflammatory drug regimen, whether it be aspirin or ibuprofen. Also, I'm now hearing rumblings that maybe aspirin doesn't help as much as previously thought, especially people who haven't previously suffered a heart attack.[9] (The medical community changing its mind? How surprising!) So do your research and talk with your doctor, who is, hopefully up to date on all the latest research.

Tomatoes and Saw Palmetto

It would appear that tomatoes contain a powerful anti-oxidant called lycopene. Tomato paste, cooked tomatoes, raw tomatoes – they all are high in lycopene, which is good for helping fight off prostate cancer, so bring on the spaghetti.

You've probably also read about the benefits of saw palmetto. Here I can give you a personal testimonial. My husband takes this regularly and at seventy-one his PSA count is low. We recently were visiting with a friend who mentioned needing to make several nocturnal visits to the bathroom due to an enlarged prostate. My husband recommended he try saw palmetto and within a couple of weeks he'd seen a marked difference. You can get this over the counter, no prescription needed. If you or someone you love is having prostate problems, this might be worth looking into.

. . .

Hormone replacement therapy

Kids, definitely don't try this on your own. This needs to be supervised by a physician who specializes in the field. Your hormone levels need to be monitored, adjustments need to be made. Hormones are powerful things and while they can do great good they can also do great harm if they're out of control.

I did natural hormone therapy for a year, and let me tell you, I slept great and didn't have any aches and pains. Woohoo! I also had trouble balancing my levels. I lasted for about a year and then decided this wasn't for me.

A couple of years or so later I wound up with uterine cancer. I honestly don't know if there was a correlation between the two. I was sure there was and asked three different specialists about that. Had I brought this on myself? They all assured me I hadn't. Still, I will always wonder. Needless to say, I've abandoned splashing around in the fountain of youth. For me, it's not worth the risk.

After researching and talking with a specialist, you may feel differently. There certainly are benefits. I would caution you to let your doctor monitor you closely though.

I know a big complaint among women after menopause is the whole vaginal dryness thing. As we age, the vaginal wall gets thinner and intercourse isn't so fun anymore. Actually, as we age and our hormone levels drop, often so does our interest in sex, which, should, theoretically, save us from having to worry about our vaginas at all. But if our husbands can still manage to work up some enthusiasm for bedroom sports, then it's game on, anyway. That leaves many women complaining that intercourse doesn't feel so good, and a lot of doctors are quick to prescribe an estrogen cream for that.

This definitely helps and I have friends who swear by it. If there is no history of cancer in your family you may want to ask your doctor about an estrogen cream for the dryness, but you might want to explore other options first. If concern over possible harmful side effects makes you nervous there are other ways around vaginal dryness that don't carry any risk. Coconut oil and a vaginal dilator to keep you moist or the use of an over the counter lubricant during intercourse will also do the trick, ladies.

Sleep Aids

I'm not talking about the prescription variety. I have no experience with those and lately what I've been reading about them has me convinced I don't want to go there.

For example, according to an article in *Medical News Today*, researchers have discovered a significant link between non-prescription sleep aids and an increased risk of dementia in older people.[10] Antihistamines containing Diphenhydramine also received a thumbs down.[11] These block the action of the neurotransmitter acetylcholine in the brain. And why, you may ask, is that a problem? Because acetylcholine is very necessary for a happy, healthy brain. This neurotransmitter helps us focus, learn, and stay mentally alert. It enhances brain plasticity. If that transmitter is blocked you are going to have memory problems.

To quote the head researcher of this particular study, Professor Shelly Gray of the University of Washington School of Pharmacy, "Older adults should be aware that many medications – including some available without a prescription such as over-the-counter sleep aids – have strong anticholinergic effects." Translation: let the sleep-deprived beware.

The good doctor did go on to advise people not to stop their therapy based on the findings of this study but to talk to their care provider and also tell the provider about all their over the counter drug use. Good advice. Say it with me, check with your doc. Always check with your doc on health-related issues.

It would appear that anti-anxiety medications, the most common of which include benzodiazepines, are not necessarily brain friendly, either. Scientists are saying these drugs are associated with a higher risk of Alzheimer's. (I don't know about you, but that's enough to make me anxious!) Here's a comforting quote from that article: "... researchers say that among 1,796 people with Alzheimer's disease and 7,184 controls, those who have used benzodiazepines showed a 51 percent higher risk of the neurodegenerative disorder. Among people who took the drugs more than 180 days, the risk escalated about two-fold higher."[12]

Now that I've about scared you to death and really depressed you, let me remind you that this was one study. Your doctor may assure you that you are perfectly fine with what you're taking.

I found that melatonin, which can be purchased over the counter, helped me sleep. This is something our bodies naturally make, but, as with many things, we produce less of it as we age. I took it for years with no adverse effects. I started with three mg then eventually started taking between five and ten, depending on what was going on. I'd start with five of the time-released variety. Then, if I woke up in the night and it looked like I wasn't going to get back to sleep, I'd take another five.

That was in the past. Dealing with a new health reality now, I've read that use of melatonin if you're on blood thinners can elevate the risk for bleeding. So, until I get my heart issues sorted out it looks like I'll be finding other ways of lulling myself to sleep at night.

One other caution regarding melatonin, if you take too much you will have strange, unsettling dreams. And, according to what I found poking around on the internet, it can cause headache, short-term feelings of depression (and then you'd be back to taking more drugs) daytime sleepiness, dizziness, stomach cramps and irritability in some people. I never personally experienced any of those, but if this leaves you leery of trying it, or, if like me, medications you're taking leave it off your list of options, you might prefer to stick to a cup of chamomile tea before bed or a nice warm bath with lavender bath salts. Or maybe we'll have to drift off to the land of Nod listening to music or audio books.

For those of us with acid reflux issues, another sleep aid to consider (if you're not on omeprazole) is taking an antacid before bedtime. That whole lying prone thing can result in acid reflux and will wake you up at night.

So will pain. One night I'd overdone it and everything ached. I took something for pain before bed and slept soundly all night. In fact, after some self-diagnosis, Dr. Sheila concluded that her sleep was often disturbed by pain. (And here I thought I was only waking up because I had to go to the bathroom!) Applying some analgesic cream or a pain patch on the problem areas has done wonders for getting my Zzz's.

If sleep is evading you, see if you can figure out what's keeping you awake or waking you up. Perhaps one of these simple solutions will solve the problem.

Stress also is a huge contributor to lack of sleep so if you're stressed or worried, talk to your doctor about possible medications that might help. St John's Wort is a tried and true ancient herb that many people find helpful, but it can interact with other drugs, so don't go running off to your local drug store to buy something without consulting a health care professional first. (A quick side note here. I recently found a page on a website that is helpful when wondering what you can and can't take if you're on a certain medication. It might be worth checking out. It's: https://www.rxlist.com/drug-interactions)

For me, one of the best stress relievers is talking about my troubles with close friends. Sometimes talking about what's bothering you rather than carrying it around lightens that load of worry. So does prayer. Same principle. I'm getting rid of that load of worry. Focusing on what's good in your life helps, too. Remember that old song about counting your blessings. There's a lot of truth in that. Find some positive sayings and quote them to yourself as you're going to sleep.

Sometimes we simply have trouble turning off our minds. If you find that to be the case work to calm your mind with some deep breathing. Or distract yourself from all those spinning thoughts by listening to something pleasant on your radio or iPad. I actually stream old-time radio programs and those voices distract me from my own whirly-gig thoughts.

Listening to something on your device and staring at your device are two different things. Being on your computer right up until bedtime will not be conducive to a good night's sleep so be sure to turn it off a couple of hours before you turn in.

Keeping your stomach in good working order also helps you sleep well, so how about a little yogurt before bed? You'll not only get those probiotics to help your insides function, but you'll also get some extra calcium.

We all feel better, function better and look better after a good night's sleep. Hopefully, if you're having sleep problems, one of these suggestions will help you get the Z's you need.

Probiotics

Here's another thing we may not have enough of as we age. An increasing number of studies are linking the health of our stomachs to our overall mental health and well-being.[13] Gas, bloating, diarrhea, constipation, heartburn – they all can be signs of trouble with the digestive system. (Gut troubles can also mess with our immune system.) Who can save our tummies and intestines from these troubles? Enter the super heroes, probiotics. In addition to keeping our gut healthy and preventing that nasty diarrhea many of us get when we take antibiotics, they can also help our hearts keep healthy. So there's more than one reason to have some yogurt before you go to bed. (Just make sure you buy the kind that actually has live cultures in it.) You can also purchase probiotic supplements specially formulated for seniors at your local health foods store.

. . .

Water and Roughage

We need both to keep everything moving. (And you may have noticed that, just like with the outside of our bodies, our insides are also moving more slowly these days.) You've heard the recommended amount of water we're supposed to drink – eight glasses a day. Remember, you can liven up the taste with sliced cucumber or chunks of honeydew melon. This last one is my personal favorite. I cut the melon into chunks, then stick them in the freezer to use as ice cubes.

As for the fiber, according to Neil Wiegand, PA-C, MCHS, who specializes in colon and rectal surgery, there's no such thing as too much fiber. Are you getting enough? Bran muffins are great and so is bran cereal. Want fast and easy? Try fiber gummies. For me, two of those in the morning and a small dose of magnesium at night is all I need to stay regular. Might work for you, too. One thing you don't want to do is be straining. A sure recipe for hemorrhoids!

And then...

It's not enough simply to eat well, exercise and supplement our diet with good things. Even the healthiest of us probably will get caught by something creepy. As we age it's important to monitor our bodies and be aware of any changes. With that in mind, here's a list of things we should all have checked on a regular basis:

Skin

As we age all kinds of spots and dots start showing up. Most of them are benign, but some are not. Get a yearly skin check-up with a dermatologist. And if you see a suspicious looking mole don't put off going in. Hypochondriac that I am, I have run to my skin doctor many a time with things that look suspicious (in fact I have an appointment in two weeks to get something checked).

This gets a little embarrassing, but she assures me that it's always better to check. Especially since I'm no expert.

Breast, Uterus, and Prostate Checks

I'm sure I don't have to tell you why it's important to get these check-ups. I've learned that after we reach the age of sixty some doctors don't feel it necessary to do a pap smear on women. Insist on it. My uterine cancer hit at the age of sixty-two, and I've talked to other older women who also had to battle the disease long after that magic number of sixty.

When I went in for my last mammogram I asked the technician how much longer I had to keep getting one. "Until you die," she replied. Breast cancer knows no age limits. She did add, however, that often older women will develop a very slow growing cancer and eventually die of other causes. Don't think I'm quite there yet, so I'll continue to visit Bertha the Boob Crusher on a yearly basis.

And men, you don't get off the hook. Have your prostate and PSA level checked regularly. Early detection is so important. (And take your saw palmetto!)

Endoscopies and Colonoscopies

If you've had extreme heartburn problems, get thee to a specialist and have your esophagus scoped to make sure you haven't developed a condition called Barrett's Esophagus. This is where you burn your poor esophagus to the point that the tissue is changed and becomes vulnerable to esophageal cancer. Once that happens you'll need to be monitored. Better to be monitored and treated than to let something like that go undiscovered.

The same holds true for colonoscopies so ask your doctor if you're due for one. If there is a history of colon cancer in your family your doctor will probably want to check you every five years instead of the standard ten.

Eyes

Regular eye check-ups are so important. As we age we're vulnerable to everything from cataracts to macular degeneration to glaucoma. Glaucoma is especially nasty as, according to my ophthalmologist, it can sneak up on you with no warning. And if it goes undetected it can lead to blindness. This is preventable, so make sure you get your eyes checked.

And, of course, a yearly check up with your general physician is a must. Staying on top of your physical and mental health will go a long way toward assuring satisfying senior living.

Social Interaction

According to an article in Forbes, a lonely person is significantly more likely to suffer an early death than a non-lonely one.[14] Researchers at Brigham Young University conducted a study and found that social isolation increases your risk of death before you're ready to go by thirty percent. If you're not planning to depart this earth yet, make sure you're interacting with others. Get out and see people, call a friend. Perhaps it's time to join a fraternal organization such as the Elks or Eagles, get involved in your local church, or take some classes through your local parks and recreation center. Check out what's happening at your local senior center. Most offer a number of activities which give seniors an opportunity to make new friends. Even if you're not an extrovert, it's worth the effort to push yourself a little outside of your comfort zone so you have some human interaction. Remember, even the Lone Ranger had Tonto.

Okay, there are my list of no-no's and yes yes's. Now, let me share advice from some of the people I interviewed for this book.

. . .

ADVICE FROM HEALTH-CONSCIOUS SENIORS

One couple I went to is Joe and Vivian Zorich, both in their eighties and still going strong. The first thing Joe advised when I asked him was, "Drink good whiskey."

But he did have more advice for those of us who aren't big drinkers, and one important bit of advice was to eat good food. Joe and Vivian eat mostly seafood and chicken, fruit and vegetables. They supplement their diet with Vitamins E, C4 and D (1,000 units a day). "Stay active," says Joe. These two are good examples of that – they both go dancing at our favorite Elks Club on a regular basis. In fact, there have been times when my husband and I left to go home to bed and Joe and Viv were still on the dance floor, kicking up their heels. Joe and Vivian also stress the importance that faith plays in their lives, as well as being involved with family.

May Sikora, at the time of this writing, is about to turn sixty-five. She and her husband moved to the southern part of the U.S., and she says she has found the warmer weather perfect for being active. She says, "An early morning walk with an open mind (and a bottle of water) turned from a one-mile walk into a ten-mile walk over an eighteen-month period. I have entered a few 5 K and 10 K races, and I just signed up for my first half marathon as a challenge before I turn sixty-five." As for watching her diet, she says she sits outside to eat her meals, which causes her to slow down and take in the scenery. "No inhaling of foods!!!" May advises "Everything in moderation… except watching the beauty in a downpour or the sun shining."

At the age of sixty-four Karen Morrell is still working full time as a middle school teacher. "Working keeps my mind sharp," she says. "Also there's no time to snack during the day." Even if there was, I suspect Karen would burn it off. She rides her exercise bike five to seven miles every night after dinner while watching the news. Karen has no intention of retiring. She can easily stay employed because she established her own school, Spring Creek Academy in Plano, Texas. And, giving Karen bragging rights here, her school numbers three gold medal Olympians among their graduates. Go Karen!

Remember Irene Lennard, our dancing queen? Here are some of her secrets for keeping healthy. She eats fresh. "I don't eat junk food and I don't eat pre-made dishes, frozen or otherwise. The only thing I eat out of a can is mackerel," she says. She's not a vegetarian, but she is big on vegetables and homemade soups, and she eats a lot of fish. "I eat to stay well," she told me. "You are what you eat." She has an alcoholic drink every day. In the winter that drink is whiskey with lemon. On a cold day, it's gin and tonic or a beer. "Guard your health and stay active," she advises. Good advice for all of us in a day when so many of us are couch potatoes.

Debbie Luchka is a big believer in working out. She recommends checking into Silver Sneakers, a program designed to encourage older adults to participate in physical activities that will help them stay healthy. It offers many stay-fit options for people over sixty-five: yoga, swimming, cardio, nutrition. This program is available around the country and membership provides access to any participating gym. It's considered a basic fitness source and, while original Medicare plans don't cover it, it would appear that Medicare Advantage plans (Medicare Part C) may.

Katrina Carlisle is sixty-five and struggles with liver disease which, she says, requires her to keep her weight in check. She doesn't eat red meat, butter or bad fats and carries tiny bottles of olive oil with her when eating away from home to use as dressing for salad or a butter substitute for a baked potato. She claims that exercise is key to keeping her weight down, so in addition to making sure she doesn't consume more than 1600 calories a day, she teaches water aerobics twice a week and rides her bicycle on weekends, riding on a sixteen-mile trail. I'd say Katrina is a good example of rising above physical challenges and maintaining a healthy lifestyle.

As these people are proving, we can maintain good health in our old age and, even when health challenges arrive, manage to deal with them.

This is all, of course, only a snapshot of the whole picture of maintaining good health, and is meant to encourage and inspire you. I would highly recommend that you get to your local library or bookstore and pick out some books by health professionals. If possible, go online and study up on what's good and what isn't, take notes, make some lifestyle changes. You're worth it.

1. John Medina, *Brain Rules for Aging Well* (Pear Press, 2017).
2. Neuro.hms.harvard.edu: *Dancing and the Brain*, Copyright 2019. http://neuro.hms.harvard.edu/harvard-mahoney-neuroscience-institute/brain-newsletter/and-brain-series/dancing-and-brain
3. Nytimes.com: *The Best Sport for a Longer Life? Try Tennis*, Copyright 2019. https://www.nytimes.com/2018/09/05/well/move/the-best-sport-for-a-longer-life-try-tennis.html?action=click&module=Discovery&pgtype=Homepage
4. Chris Crowley and Henry S. Lodge, M.D., *Younger Next Year* (Workman Publishing, 2004).
5. Heart.harvard.edu: *The Sweet Danger of Sugar*, Copyright 2019. https://www.health.harvard.edu/heart-health/the-sweet-danger-of-sugar
6. Heart.org: *Saturated Fat*, Copyright 2019.

HTTP://WWW.HEART.ORG/EN/HEALTHY-LIVING/HEALTHY-EATING/EAT-SMART/FATS/SATURATED-FATS

1. Rebecca Katz and Mat Edelson, *The Healthy Mind Cookbook* (Berkley, Ten Speed Press, 2015).
2. Michael E. Roizen, M.D., *Real Age: Are You as Young as You Can Be?* (Harper Collins, 1999).
3. Healthline.com: *Taking an Aspirin a Day to Prevent Heart Attack or Stroke May be Risky*, Copyright 2019.

https://www.healthline.com/health-news/aspirin-heart-attack-stroke-050614#1

1. Medicalnewstoday.com: *Over-the-Counter Sleeps Aids Linked to Dementia*, Copyright 2019.

https://www.medicalnewstoday.com/articles/288546.php

1. Cbsnews.com: *Popular Drugs for Colds Allergies Linked to Dementia*, Copyright 2019.

https://www.cbsnews.com/news/popular-drugs-for-colds-allergies-linked-to-dementia/

1. Time.com: *Alzheimer's Linked to Sleeping Pills and Anti-Anxiety Drugs*, Copyright 2019.

http://time.com/3313927/alzheimers-linked-to-sleeping-pills-and-anti-anxiety-drugs/

1. Healthline.com: 8 Benefits of Probiotics, Copyright 2019.

https://www.healthline.com/nutrition/8-health-benefits-of-probiotics#section3

1. Forbes.com: *Loneliness Might be a Bigger Health Risk than Smoking or Obesity*, Copyright 2017.

https://www.forbes.com/sites/quora/2017/01/18/loneliness-might-be-a-bigger-health-risk-than-smoking-or-obesity/#26c4363425d1

6. WHAT NOW, MY LOVE? LIFESTYLE CHANGES AND CHALLENGES

At this point in our journey we've all learned that life is full of change. I always say that I'm not that fond of change... unless it's good and it's happening to me.

Those changes that deprive us of the quality of life we've enjoyed in the past can be especially unsettling. This last summer a bout of tendinopathy took me off the tennis courts for a month. In August. The month I'd planned on playing three times a week with my beach pals. Oh, the agony. And before that it was the torn rotator cuff. Sheesh. I wound up trying to teach myself how to play left-handed. That was a scene worthy of an *I Love Lucy* episode!

Has something like that happened to you? Maybe even on a larger scale? Have you had to say a permanent good-bye to a sport or hobby you love? Have you had to radically alter your lifestyle? How difficult that is!

But don't despair. I'm sure you've heard the saying, that which doesn't kill me makes me stronger. Or how about this one? When one door closes another one opens.

You may be thinking, *Thanks for that dose of triteness, and now I'd like to close a door in your face, Sheila. Or on it. You have no idea what I'm going through.*

You're right, I don't. But let me see if I can encourage you with some inspiration and advice from others who have faced or are still dealing with physical challenges. My hope is that these real-life stories will encourage you.

I recently interviewed a lovely woman named Pat, who had to completely leave behind the game of tennis when rheumatoid arthritis hit her, making it too painful to play. She was sixty-one. The symptoms first appeared when she was on the court and she said to her teammate, "I hurt from one end to the other." She found a doctor who was able to help her feel better, but her days on the court were still over.

She didn't spend too much time mourning the loss of her game. A neighbor down the road was offering a painting class and she decided to attend. Pat says that was the beginning of a whole new life. She not only found a new hobby, she found a new set of friends.

She's now been painting for twenty years, has participated in art shows and sold many paintings. Still, tennis... Having played the game since I was thirteen, hearing her story made me shudder.

I asked Pat if it was hard to let go of doing something she loved and she replied, "I was so busy with other things I didn't have time to think about it. I don't sit around and mope." Her advice is, "If you have to give up one thing find something else immediately."

Pat also recommends cultivating younger friends. She went younger because her old friends were "getting so boring." At eighty-one Pat is definitely not a boring woman. And she doesn't lack for friends. "Groups are wonderful," she says.

If you're encountering roadblocks to certain activities, I encourage you to find ways around them. And meanwhile, try to encourage yourself by using the tried and true method of looking on the bright side. Yes, it can (not always, but often) be worse.

Sometimes, it can also get better. And sometimes getting to better takes a great deal of commitment and dedication.

One of my much-loved family members, Clay Moyle, is entering his sixties still dealing with the side effects of something that happened to him when he was fifty-eight. He fell off a ladder and suffered a third-grade concussion, a.k.a. mild-traumatic brain injury (TBI). "To say the injury turned my whole world upside down would be putting it mildly," Clay told me. "It's not called a 'traumatic' brain injury for nothing." His injury caused blurred and double vision for the next year, along with a host of cognitive issues for the following three.

Clay is one determined man though and he did a massive amount of research about his particular condition. His persistence paid off and he was able to finally overcome the visual problems that resulted from this injury after finding and working with a neuro-optometrist. He's still working with a specialist on a couple of issues.

I talked with Clay and also read a series of articles he wrote about his experience. Here is a quote from one of them which I found inspiring and hope you will, too. "Time, rest and patience are key, but I've learned there are specific actions one can take to aid their own recovery in terms of both the rate and degree of that recovery. I'm determined to do everything I possibly can to realize a complete recovery as quickly as I possibly can.[1]

"As a result of my own research, I learned that while most parties realize a full recovery from a mild TBI within six months it can often take as long as a year for those of us over the age of forty. I couldn't imagine enduring the personal hell I was going through the first couple of months for as long as six months, let alone a year, but once I accepted the facts and I settled in for a much longer ride than originally anticipated," Clay said.

When I asked his advice for someone dealing with healing from a traumatic injury he replied, "Become your own best advocate."

He first went to a well-respected clinic associated with a prestigious university but didn't get much help beyond a diagnosis, a prescription for anxiety medication and a suggestion that he work with one of their psychologists who they promised would give him the tools to deal with his new reality. His new reality included sensitivity to light, brain fog, dizziness, and extreme fatigue on top of the vision issues.

"Online research and networking gave me an opportunity to learn and share experiences with others who were either suffering or had suffered from something similar."

Clay makes a good point about networking. Sometimes our friends, even our own family can't understand or empathize with what we're going through. Find others who are dealing with the same issues you are so you can get much-needed emotional and spiritual support. There are many support groups online to help people dealing with health conditions and other life challenges.

Clay adds, "I really did put my trust in the Lord. I prayed every day that he'd light the path to follow and believed the steps I followed along the way were that path. I prayed for the strength, courage and faith to diligently follow it each morning."

When we encounter what look like dead ends on the road back to our normal life it's important to do everything we possibly can to get where we want to go. Those dead ends could simply be detours. But if they turn out to be insurmountable, then we need to be open to exploring new destinations.

Finding our way back to normal, whether it's the old, familiar normal or a new normal, isn't always pleasant. So, how to cope?

Sometimes it helps to vent. Linda Theriault is a breast cancer survivor. However, she's still dealing with MS, fibromyalgia and diabetes. "Right now my balance is sooo off I wall walk (hands along the walls everywhere)!" she told me. "Annoying!"

Annoying? That's an understatement. She copes with her troubles by allowing herself a five minute rant/pity party every day. She believes that sometimes you just have to get that unhappiness out of your system. After the pity party, it's back to concentrating on what's good in her life, her grandson. "Bad day + phone call from Damien = complete turn-around for me!" she says.

Dawna Penrod suffers from rheumatoid arthritis. She's had both knees replaced and is now on oxygen 24/7 due to the ravages of the disease on her lungs. She took disease modifying IV's once a month for many years that made the pain more tolerable but now, due to the issue with her lungs, she's no longer able to.

Dawna says, "There are two pearls of wisdom that keep me going with a positive outlook. Pain is inevitable but misery is optional. And, 'Do not let what you cannot do interfere with what you CAN do,' a quote by John Wooden." Good advice Dawna!

Nancy McCoy's husband was diagnosed in the fall of 2013 with idiopathic pulmonary fibrosis. He went on oxygen in October of 2014, and by February of 2015 received a bilateral lung transplant. He had to retire early from his job as a school principal and Nancy had to quit work to become his caregiver.

"Our lifestyle has changed drastically," she told me, "but our faith has sustained us." In addition to staying strong spiritually, Nancy and her husband took practical steps, moving to be closer to both doctors and family.

As of this writing, one of my beach buddies, Mary Harms is bracing for surgery on her left foot for posterior tibial tendon insufficiency stage three (or, in layman's terms, advanced flat foot deformity). They will stabilize four joints in her left foot, then after six weeks they will operate on her right foot. It means months in a wheelchair for this active lady.

"I was shocked at first," Mary told me. "It left me in a puddle of tears. But God is good, and He will be with me, along with the prayers of so many friends and family." Mary is preparing physically for her upcoming ordeal, working on getting in shape by water walking. She's worked up to an hour in the pool and goes three times a week. She also plans to cook a few meals ahead of time. I suspect she'll wind up with more meals than she can eat once all her friends start pitching in.

Which brings me to some practical advice of my own. If you're adjusting to a new life with physical challenges, don't be afraid to ask for help where you need it.

Men often let their pride get in the way of asking for assistance. Guys, we know that you're strong and tough and capable, but once in a while it's okay to take time off from being strong and tough. Get help now so you can go back to being self-sufficient later.

And ladies, yes, we are normally givers and it can feel uncomfortable to be on the receiving end of help. When I was undergoing chemo, my friends became an army of helpers – vacuuming, bringing food, hiring someone to put our lawn and garden in shape, or simply coming to Sheila-sit and keep me company. There were times when I felt like a leech. But I came to realize that my friends wanted to help me and being of use was as good for them as their assistance was for me. We all experience an emotional lift when we do good for others. So let your friends help you so they can feel good about themselves.

Determination plays a big part in how well we overcome obstacles. Facebook friend, Karen Oram-Proudfoot, endured back surgery, a severe infection that almost killed her and a second surgery. Karen wound up in an inpatient rehab facility for four months. "I didn't want to remain wheelchair bound and I tried sooo hard to get back my life!" She did. "I walk on my own without assistance and keep on rolling," says Karen. Obviously, without the wheelchair. She shared that her husband wasn't as motivated when he had an issue to deal with and still needs to use a walker.

It's easier to keep that determination if you have a goal to work for. In Karen's case it was being able to walk again. For Clay it was getting back into top physical condition so he could once more play basketball. For my friend Pat's husband, who is battling cancer for a second time, that goal is getting back on the tennis court. He talks a lot about returning to tennis, which keeps that goal firmly in front of him.

What is your goal? Do you have a dream yet to be fulfilled? Perhaps reminding yourself of it on a regular basis will help you as you work toward conquering difficult challenges.

Remember though, if a door on one part of your life closes, start looking for the door that will lead you in a new direction. Keep in mind the story of Pat, who went from tennis to painting and remember that giving up one thing doesn't mean giving up everything.

Right now I'm having to remind myself of that. I had stem cell therapy scheduled for my knees until the night I wound up in the emergency room with atrial fibrillation. Only three days before I was supposed to stop use of any and all blood-thinning anti-inflammatory drugs such as aspirin and ibuprofen for a week, I wound up coming home with – you guessed it – a prescription for blood thinners. Atrial fibrillation, blood clots, and stroke appear to go hand in hand. So good-bye new knees.

As soon as the doctor left my husband and me alone with my heart monitor, I threw myself a huge pity party and had a good cry. Seriously? This had to happen a week before my knee patch job?

I'm still working on adjusting my attitude. One thing that helps with the adjustment is reminding myself to be thankful this happened before I had the procedure done. What if my heart had acted up later and I wound up on these blood-thinning meds? After stem-cell replacement therapy you can't take so much as an aspirin for six weeks. And, according to the nurse I whined to, you do have to be off blood thinners for a couple days during all this. I'd have undone everything that had been done and spent thousands of dollars (as of this writing my insurance doesn't cover regenerative medicine) for nothing. So, as we explore future options, I keep reminding myself to look at the silver lining in this particular cloud and to keep my health priorities straight. Heart and brain before knees! And I'm determined to be thankful for modern medicine and the fact that, thanks to this medication, my frisky heart is getting reined in. As of this writing I'm looking into various repair options and telling my knees, "Suck it up and get in line."

If your plans just got tossed out the window, I encourage you to try and get in touch with your inner Pollyanna – remember her from that old Disney movie? – and play the glad game. What can you still be glad about? What can you be thankful for? I believe it's important to find something. Otherwise, misery becomes your new best friend.

Perhaps you're having to reinvent your lifestyle. If so, ask yourself, "What new area do I now have a chance to explore?" And fill in the blanks on this question: If I can't ________, can I ________?

Looking for new possibilities and opportunities can turn our focus in a more positive direction. Perhaps you aren't going to be able to be as physically active as previously. Will that give you more time to exercise your brain and enjoy activities such as reading or writing? If a health challenge is turning you in a new direction maybe part of that new direction will be sharing your story with others and offering tips on how to cope. Perhaps you'll start writing magazine articles or speaking to service clubs or church groups. Be on the lookout for new opportunities, new challenges, and new adventures.

I Can Do It Myself … Or Not

Another change most of us don't like to accept is that of giving up our independence. After all, we've been independent for many years, making our own decisions, running our own lives. Which is probably why it comes as a shock when we realize we can't quite do the things we did twenty, ten, or maybe even two years ago.

This lifestyle constriction can take many forms – having to hire someone to do the yard work we once enjoyed, perhaps opting for assisted living or, the other biggie so many of us dread, giving up the luxury of driving. But when it's time, it's time.

Baby, You Can Drive My Car

Let's start by talking about that love affair most of us have with our cars. Let's face it, there will come a time when that relationship must come to an end. As we age, our eyesight fails, our hearing fades, and our reflexes slow down. That can prove dangerous, not only to ourselves but to others on the road as well.

Recently when I was at the post office I watched in horror as an elderly man slooowly got behind the wheel of his car. I've seen turtles move faster. I couldn't help asking myself what would happen if this man had to suddenly stop his vehicle.

I still remember vividly the last time I went somewhere with my mother in her car. She seemed to have suddenly lost the concept of yielding to oncoming traffic when making a left-hand turn at a traffic signal. Three times in a row I had to alert her to an oncoming car. Shortly after that, we found a way to diplomatically separate Mom from her vehicle. One of her friends, however, didn't give up driving until she got in a small accident. Happily, she realized that for her, too, the time had come, and graciously relinquished her driving privileges.

Not so my elderly father-in-law. He was a great guy and a lousy driver. And determined to keep his driver's license to the bitter end. Thankfully, he managed to do so without taking out any of the other drivers on the road. Instead, he merely terrified my mother-in-law every time they drove somewhere together. (Not to mention worrying his kids.)

According to one study I read, people over sixty-five are

sixteen percent more likely than other adult drivers to have an accident.[2] If it's any consolation though, much younger drivers (fifteen to twenty-four) are one-hundred and eighty-eight times more likely than us to cause an accident. Now, before you go getting cocky let me also point out that older drivers are more breakable. In an accident, one of us older people is five-hundred and seventy percent more likely to be killed than our younger versions.

If your reflexes are still good and you're careful about when and where you drive, you're probably fine, especially if you invest in a new vehicle that comes with safety features like blind spot detection, automatic braking, and lane departure warning. But if your eyesight and hearing are failing, if you're starting to have serious health issues, if you're not as focused as you once were, think twice about taking any long car trips. I still shudder thinking about one of our friends who recently had a mini-stroke while driving and started seeing double. Happily, he was able to pull off the road and let his wife take the wheel. But what if he'd been alone? What if you're alone and that happens? Don't put your children in the painful position of having to take your car keys from you. Or worse, having to rush to the emergency room to see you. (We want our kids to visit us, but not there!)

Instead, plan for how you can manage to get where you want to go to get what you need. These days, grocery stores deliver and we can shop on line or call Uber or a taxi or take a bus, a train or a plane. We can carpool. We have options. Admit when it's time to exchange that driver's license for other ways of getting from here to there and try to do it with good grace. Console yourself with the thought that you might be saving someone's life. Like yours.

Living Situations

Chances are there will come a time when your living arrangements have to change. This brings its own unique stress. Do you do from a two-level home to a rambler? Do you downsize? If so, how much? What do you keep? What do you get rid of? Where should you live? Do you live near your kids? With them? Away from them? What if your kids all live in different parts of the country? Who do you pick to live near? What if none of your offspring are inclined to help you? What if you don't have kids?

Let's try and break this down, one issue at a time.

Move or Stay Put?

Of course, the first consideration when deciding whether you can stay in your home or not is, how capable are you of living independently? Are you still able to cook and clean for yourself? If cooking has become a challenge, do you have access to a program that will deliver meals to you? Are you near a family member who is willing to assist you with big tasks that might require more stamina than you have? Can you afford to hire help with yard work and cleaning?

If the answer to all that is yes, then you're good to go. Stay in your home or get a slightly smaller one with less square footage to clean and less yard to maintain. Or you might want to purchase a condo where you have access to community. (And elevators!) If, however, you're facing physical challenges then you'll need to consider either moving in with one of your offspring or finding an assisted living facility.

If you have more than one child, picking who to live with or near can be a challenge. If you have a good relationship with all your kids, you may need to call a family meeting to discuss possibilities.

Diplomacy is important. We have a son and a daughter, both of whom we dearly love and enjoy. Our son and his wife put in a bid early to take care of us in our old age. Actually, this sounded smart. Even though my daughter and I are best friends and have a great time together, our styles are very different and we have joked many a time that if we lived together we'd kill each other. However, when I told her that it looked like her brother had drawn the short end of the stick and was going to be taking care of us in our old age she quipped, "Who said he gets to have the short end of the stick?" (Gotta love that girl.) Even though I think her feelings might have been a little hurt (as were mine when my mom chose to leave her home next door to us and move to a nearby town with my big brother), I'm glad this got settled. We're not there yet. (In fact, we hope never to get there.) But if the time comes, hopefully, all concerned will experience less frustration.

One thing I don't want to be, and that's stubborn. If I reach a point where I need to relocate then I hope I can do so with grace, just as my own mother did. Remaining independent is important to our self-esteem, but we don't want to boost that at the cost of making life difficult for the ones who are watching over us.

I still remember my mother and father-in-law in their late eighties insisting on remaining independent. Well, they sort of were. Unless one of them had to go into the hospital. Then one of us would go stay with the one who remained at home. We also made regular trips to the house to help with housecleaning and handyman chores. This was a bit of a trek, as they'd picked their dream home far from most of their adult children. So, independent? More like semi-independent.

Having said that, I should point out that no one minded helping. We loved them. Maybe your children won't mind helping you a lot, either.

Or maybe you'll become one more thing on a long to-do list as they juggle their own parental obligations and work schedules. It's a good idea to carefully assess your circumstances and make sure your independence isn't coming at too high a cost for your adult children.

If you're planning to remain independent you'd better know exactly how that will look. Make sure any family members who will be impacted by your decision are on board with it and really will be able to help you when you need it. That old joke about living to be a burden to your children isn't so funny when it becomes a reality.

Moving in with our kids can be a win-win for all. It was for my family when my grandmother lived with us. But it can also prove stressful. Try some extended visits to see how well you cope with each other's schedules and daily habits before committing to something permanent. You might mesh beautifully, but if you don't, the time to find out is before the moving truck pulls away.

If you feel living under the same roof will make for too much togetherness consider going in together on a house that includes separate living quarters for you such as a mother-in-law apartment or guest wing or purchasing a duplex where you can live side by side. Or move nearby. We wound up purchasing a condo that's ten minutes away from our son and his daughter. Not much maintenance required (hopefully), and we have the benefit of enjoying each other's company while still giving our adult children some space.

The younger generation moves a lot more than we or our parents did. If that's the case in your family this may not be the way to go. Instead, you may need to consider alternative living arrangements.

If there is no younger generation in your life, you definitely will need to be your own advocate. If you're planning to remain in your home, make sure you have what you need to stay safe, such as grab bars next to the toilet and in the shower. You might also want to invest in a comfort height toilet, which sits at a higher level and is much easier on the knees. Taking advantage of voice activated technology that can help you remember appointments, birthdays and when to take medications. And make friends with your neighbors. Not knowing the people you live next to will only serve to isolate you. On the other hand, if you interact with the people around you, you have some sort of security net.

A roommate provides companionship and shares expenses and chores. The ideal would be to find someone a little younger (and more fit and agile) than you who shares your interests. Remember the old TV show *The Golden Girls*? Sounds like fun to me!

You can also look into joining a village. The Village to Village network is an organization that supplies support, resources, and expert advice for people wanting to come together and live communally. This organization's vision is to expand opportunities and support for older people. It will most likely be a more affordable option than assisted living.

Assisted Living

This is a good option if you're alone. It's also a good choice if you want to stay close to your roots or if you or your spouse is failing, either physically or mentally. Meals and cleaning are taken care of, you're living in a community, and you have skilled caregivers watching over you.

Do your research before signing on the dotted line as each facility is different. Some you buy into and then are taken care of for life. These can be pricey and the company or organization running them will want to know what assets you have in addition to the money you'll be forking over initially. Some facilities will charge you monthly rent, which means you'll be good to go as long as you can pay the rent. When you can't it will be, "Adios, amigo." In addition to comparison shopping to make sure you find the facility that will be the best fit for you, it's a good idea to take someone with you when checking out possible residences so you can get an unbiased opinion and have a sounding board.

Money is, of course, another consideration. If you purchased long term care insurance then you're probably good to go. (No one likes those high premiums, but they are cheaper than the care itself.) If not, you'll have to self-insure, which can become problematic for those of us who are no longer working. Usually, this kind of change is funded by selling property. (Another reason to not get a reverse mortgage if you can help it.)

According to my friend Peggy Doviak, author of *52 Weeks to Prosperity*[3], retirement center living can get pricey. As of this writing, in her state of Oklahoma this option can eat up $250,000. (This calculation is based on the average length of stay in a care facility, which is three years.) To get an idea of what's available in your area check out interactive websites. As of this writing, a good one is https://www.seniorliving.org/lifestyles/nursing-homes/costs/

Another option is home agency care, which can run $250 a day or more. (Nursing care and memory care can run even higher.) Peggy suggests considering the private duty option, which involves not using an agency and can be significantly less expensive as there's no agency overhead. Of course, if you go this route, you (or your offspring) need to get references, check licensing, and run the caregiver's information through a criminal database.

I have often heard elder law attorney Rajiv Nagaich talk about aging issues on his Seattle radio program. He stresses the importance of working these things out ahead of time. Who will be helping you when the time comes that you need that help? Get it settled now.

Where to Live... the Rest of the Year

Have you just bought the vacation home of your dreams? Are you preparing to be a snowbird? This happy but huge change brings its own unique set of questions. How do you furnish the second place? What do you take with you? How do you handle mail? What will you do for transportation when you're there?

I suggest making a checklist so you don't lose track of what you need to do. Also, be practical. If you have things to take to the new digs consider how you are going to transport them.

My husband and I had to deal with this last question after we purchased snowbird digs near our California kids. We needed a car in sunny CA, so Gerhardt decided to drive one down and leave it there. We packed our pre-owned Volvo station wagon to the roof with dishes, pots and pans, and a chair (all garage sale and thrift store finds – the only way to furnish snowbird digs) and set off.

I'd like to say our trip was lovely and relaxing. It wasn't. It was the car trip equivalent of a forced march. Stressful and exhausting. Many sections of the Interstate we drove were in terrible condition and with every bump I was sure my dishes, which I should have packed better, were going to break. (*Someone* didn't think that through very carefully when she was organizing things.) Two different times other drivers didn't see us and came into our lane, nearly taking us out, and I strongly suspect that the first one to see catastrophe coming was little, old, panicked me and not my other half, who was behind the wheel.

We still have some furniture to transport and I'm hoping next time around we can pay someone to drive a U-Haul down for us. (Yes, we are reaching the point in life when road trips aren't a good option, and I'm more than willing to admit it!) If you're shuffling around possessions, perhaps enlisting help or hiring professionals will be a wise choice for you as well.

So might getting rid of some of that stuff if you're getting ready to relocate. I'm not saying you have to chuck everything that's necessary or pretty or has sentimental value, but I am saying it's a good idea to reduce the amount of flotsam and jetsam kicking around your house. Do you really want to move all those books and the sports equipment you no longer use, the dresses you bought on sale and never wore, that espresso maker you haven't used in the last five years? Downsizing means smaller, as in less room for everything, especially if you're going to an assisted living facility. Chances are something will have to go. Maybe even several somethings.

What can get donated to your local charity thrift store? What sentimental item might one of your family members enjoy using right now? Gift it and get it gone. For example, that set of Christmas dishes you don't use now that someone else is hosting Christmas Eve might make a perfect present for a daughter or granddaughter. Get rid of broken jewelry, outdated technology, clothes you no longer wear, extra plastic bags and expired medicine and food items.

Lightening your load will free you up to move into the next phase of your life, whatever that may look like.

And you know there will be a next phase. Life is not static. Those of us who are able to adapt and take the new curves in the road have a much better journey than those of us who don't. So, let's be flexible. Let's adapt. Let's stay ready for whatever may be around that curve.

1. Clay Moyle, *Moyle: My Post-Concussion Journey Reaches Month Nine and I'm Getting Closer to Full Recovery*, May 11, 2016. http://www.sportspaper.org/?p=2261
2. https://www.rand.org/pubs/research_briefs/RB9272.html
3. Peggy Doviak, *52 Weeks to Prosperity* (The Road Runner Press, 2018).

7. LIFE AFTER DEATH: COPING WITH LOSS

I think the worst thing about aging is reaching a point in life where, one by one, we start having to part with loved ones. Facing death is a huge, heartbreaking challenge.

Obviously, I can't give you every answer you need on how to cope with this kind of loss in only one chapter, any more than I can address every health or finance-related question. (I couldn't give it to you in one book!) But I hope I, and some of the many people I polled, can spark some thought, encourage you, and share some resources that will help you if you're dealing with loss.

Let's start with the challenge of preparing for it. If you and your spouse are still both alive, you've been granted time to ready yourselves somewhat. You can figure out how you each want to be taken care of after death. That alone is a big decision. Do you prefer burial or cremation? What kind of service do you want? You have the opportunity to make sure the will is in order and that the one of you left behind knows where all the important papers are and what gets paid to whom and when. Do each one of you have the tools you need to deal with all those everyday details without your partner by your side?

I'd love to be able to say my husband and I are completely

ready for the time when one of us goes, but I have to confess that we're not there yet. My other half can make tacos and toast and peanut butter sandwiches and that's about it. And when it comes to finances, I'm a throwback to the fifties – happy to let him handle the money, both for my business and our personal life. I manage my household money and the grocery money and that's it. To his credit, Gerhardt has made me an extensive list of where our various funds come from and who gets paid when, but to me it's like reading Greek. I keep suggesting (okay, nagging) that when it's time for bills to be paid we sit down together so I can start getting the knack of this, but so far we haven't done it. We still need to update our will, and we need to consult an expert on how to make sure profits from anything of mine published posthumously gets handled. In short, we have work to do. As of this writing it's at the top of the to-do list. Mine, anyway.

How about you? Have you talked about final wishes and final details, not only with your spouse but also with your children so you can avoid death-bed drama and fights in the hospital room? Do you know where the will is? The key to the safe deposit box? The title to the house, the car, the truck? And, on another note, do you have a support network of family or friends to help you as you deal with the trauma that accompanies death?

Most of us don't enjoy considering our own mortality, and facing that inevitability is nothing anyone looks forward to. My husband and I were no exception. Several years back, when I was undergoing chemo for uterine cancer, I called two different cemeteries to get quotes on burial plots. I was ready to go shopping. Gerhardt balked, not wanting to deal with anything beyond what was already on our plate. Then I recovered and life went on. Sadly, we did finally have to deal with this when our oldest daughter died. We not only bought a plot for her but one for each of us as well, one on either side of hers. It was horrible letting her go and having to make the funeral arrangements. Having to get burial plots on top of that was one more awful detail to have to deal with. And quickly, which added stress. So let me encourage you to learn from us and, if you have time, settle some of the business of dying right now while you're alive. It won't ease your grief but it probably will reduce your stress.

No matter how well prepared we are, it's painful to say goodbye. You may be the type of person who can power through and make all the necessary arrangements. If you're not, get help. Allow one of your children or siblings or a close friend to be your wingman as you work through the check list of everything that has to be done. You don't have to do it all. If you can't face writing the obituary get someone else to do it. Let younger family members email and call and put out the word on Facebook as to where and when the memorial service or celebration of life will be held.

When we lost my mother, my oldest brother and I went together to the funeral home to make arrangements. I wrote the obituary. My other brother handled the rest of the details of her estate. When our daughter died, I planned the memorial service, picking out songs and the order of service, but I didn't have to worry about food. Dear friends at church stepped in and took care of that. A close friend read a tribute and big brother Ben gave a eulogy. My husband and I picked out her final outfit and the coffin together. Being together helped us stay strong enough emotionally to make the needed arrangements.

If you've lost a spouse or family member, the loss hurts like it's yours alone. But usually it isn't. That sibling was a parent or friend or favored aunt or uncle. Your spouse was a parent or sibling or childhood friend. We all feel our own pain, but it is usually shared by others. Sharing the grief and the resulting burdens can be helpful for everyone concerned. I think this is why we have memorial services, funerals, celebrations of life – so that we can all comfort each other. Knowing that others appreciated your husband or wife and love and care for you can be good medicine.

Some of us would prefer to be left alone while others of us want to be surrounded by people. According to Dr. Louis E. Lagrand, author of *Healing Grief, Finding Peace:101 Ways to Cope with the Death of Your Loved One*[1], we all have a grieving style. We all choose our own unique paths to healing. And yes, the goal is to heal – but how long that takes and what it looks like will vary. There is no one right way to grieve. You may prefer to have a large service or a quiet family gathering or nothing at all. You may prefer to wait a while to have a celebration of life service until you've had a chance to process your loss somewhat. Or to give others a chance to join you. Often, if a family loses a loved one close to the holidays the family will postpone the service so it doesn't get lost in the busyness of holiday trips and celebrations. Your grieving needs to happen on your time and on your terms, no one else's. Take as much time as you need.

We all process this difficult experience differently. One of my readers, Deborah Juliano Joy, shared with me that when her father died her mother was lost. She said she would often stop by the house and find her mom sitting on the couch with her father's picture on her lap, having a full-blown conversation with him. "I told her it was OK – whatever got her through the day!" Deborah said.

Rosi Hoak told me, "I had my husband cremated and talked to his ashes on the dresser. Just like before he still didn't answer. The only reason he wasn't late to his own funeral was because someone else was driving," she added. Obviously, Rosi has been able to lighten her grief with humor. Do you have some funny anecdotes, amusing remembrances? Share them with others.

Many times we feel our spouses are still there, watching over us. Some women have even told me they saw their husbands after death – going around a corner, standing at the foot of the bed – and found it comforting. (I would find it terrifying and I hope if my other half goes first that he won't do that to me.) Perhaps you've had a similar experience. Perhaps you find comfort visiting a graveside or holding a picture or looking at old pictures with another family member. Remembering is allowed. So is being thankful for the time you had together.

You may be having trouble sleeping or find yourself unable to pull out of depression. Talk with your doctor. One of my friends, on losing her husband, gave herself permission to get a prescription for a mild anti-depressant to help her over the rough spots. I'm a crier. With each loss of someone important to me I've shed copious tears. I'm also a talker, so I've talked a lot with friends and family. Both have proved to be good therapy for me.

Probably not as good as my habit of self-medicating with food. Being a sugar addict, goodies were my drug of choice and when I lost my mother I'm sure I consumed my weight in chocolate. My father died on Good Friday. We won't even talk about how many bags of chocolate Robin's Eggs I gobbled. On the way to see my brother in the hospital after his stroke I stopped by the local grocery store and bought a chunk of cake, figuring I'd dole it out to myself over the next couple of days. By the time I got to the hospital it was gone. The comfort food thing was probably not the best coping mechanism as I then had to work later at shedding that poundage.

If you're worried about abusing drugs or alcohol, allow family or friends to set a watch over you. Have someone stay with you for a few days or go to a relative's house. Take advantage of the emotional support offered by organizations such as Alcoholics Anonymous. Don't delay. If you prefer to be alone, keep your house safe. Don't bring any substance into your house that's not doctor prescribed and can take you to a dark place. Where you are is already dark enough.

Another reader, Kathleen Bylsma told me, "Remember, the first year post-demise will be filled with the busyness of dying – all the paperwork, etc. ... the reality hits after that. Have your support system in place."

Good advice. Perhaps you can ease into positive activities to help yourself cope: getting together with friends, watching favorite TV shows, attending church services, getting involved in some sort of physical activity such as swimming or walking. Yes, allow yourself to grieve and feel that loss, but also give yourself permission to take a break from it. Whatever works with your style and temperament, do it.

At some point, consider easing into some sort of volunteer work. Taking our focus off ourselves and our own misery is often key to lifting our spirits and reminding us that we're still here for a reason. After her husband died, in addition to working, Meryle Wilson says she began visiting people who were shut-ins or in rehab after surgery. She says that really pulled her through.

Having a faith to cling to in times of loss is, in my opinion, invaluable. Revelation 14:13, the NIV translation, is a Bible verse that comforts me when I think of the family members I've lost. It also encourages me when I think about my own departure date: "...Blessed are the dead who die in the Lord from now on... they will rest from their labor, for their deeds will follow them."

When we lost our daughter it was a comfort to know that she truly was better off. She'd been severely handicapped all her life, never able to talk, run, go to school and learn, or have a career or family. No deeds there. Just a smiling face and a sweet laugh. Yet after she died, I saw her in a dream. She was sitting up in her wheelchair, with no need of assistance or a body brace, feeding herself and smiling at me. She looked like a normal child. To this day I believe that dream was a gift from God, sent to comfort me. I believe I'll see her again one day, along with the other precious family members I've lost, and this gives me hope and takes the edge off the grief. I still feel their loss. I still tear up. I still miss my big brother. And it was a year after my mother died before I could think of her without crying. But those moments of grief have become fewer and farther apart. Hopefully, that will happen for you, too, because the living still demand our attention.

Death is a horrible thing, but so are disease and suffering. If your loved one has been suffering, death can be a release. If you've been in the draining position of serving as caregiver for a long period of time death can be a release for both of you. And if, mixed with your sorrow, you also feel as if a burden has been lifted after that loved one is gone, don't feel guilty. You have gone through rough waters and survived. Now you're on the bank and you can give yourself permission to lay back, rest in the sun and regain your strength.

Sometimes we experience guilt after loss because we think we haven't done enough for the other person in life. *I should have been more patient with him... I shouldn't have made such a squawk when she wanted to redo the kitchen... We should have taken that trip... I could have been a better wife, better husband, better sister, mother, brother, child.*

I certainly had guilty thoughts after losing our daughter. I beat myself for not keeping her home her entire life, for putting her in a group home. I thought of a million ways I could have been a better mother. This was not even remotely productive. She was gone, and the past was in the past. I hadn't been perfect, but I'd tried my best at the time. I had to let it go at that.

You may have to let go of the things you haven't done right, too. If this is problematic for you, take some time and write a letter to that loved one, sharing your heart and apologizing for whatever wrongs are haunting you. Or speak the words out loud. Get it off your chest and then commit those regrets and past mistakes to the past. Bury them and leave them there. Know that your loved one is now in a place where past hurts have been left behind, where, in the light of eternity, concerns of the world are inconsequential and gone. Allow yourself to get over it. And if this is too big a project to tackle alone, set up an appointment with a grief counselor who can help you work through your pain.

Also, there are a number of websites you might find helpful. The Masters in Counseling.org website (https://www.mastersincounseling.org/guide/loss-grief-bereavement/), for example, lists a number of websites you can visit for specific help. You may want to reach out to someone in your church or synagogue to see if there is a support group you can join. Who knows? You may want to start one.

Or you may feel the need to get away from the memories. Whether you stay put or find a new locale to begin a new life is also up to you. Most experts suggest you wait a year before making any life-changing decision such as selling your house or moving, but that doesn't mean you have to lock yourself in your house for a year. I know of one woman who, rather than stay home her first Christmas without her husband, took a holiday cruise with a friend. She found stepping away from fresh wounds and putting herself in an altogether different environment immensely helpful.

Our animals can play a big part in our lives during a time of loss. Paula Eykelhof, who was my editor at my publishing house for many years and still remains a good friend, pointed this out to me. She learned this firsthand after the loss of her husband. I asked her to write down and share her thoughts on this subject. She did so eloquently and I want to share them with you.

"Animals give love and comfort—and they need it, ask for it, too. Both the giving and receiving of love help us in times of grief.

"We suffer when our animal companions do, but make no mistake: *they* also suffer on *our* behalf. Anyone with exposure to animals has experienced or at least seen it. There are numerous examples, including the well-documented grief of elephants at the death of one of their own and recently the orca whale who could not release the body of her dead baby. In my personal experience, when our dog Asta died abruptly of an aneurysm years ago, our cat Patience—who adored this dog – howled inconsolably. I (of course) burst into tears. Again.

"But what I'm addressing here is primarily the role of our animals in the case of human loss. The loss of one of us. Of *their* people.

"My husband died almost three years ago of cancer, after 2 ½ years of debilitating treatments—surgeries, endless tests, chemo, radiation. In the last year especially, he wasn't very mobile and spent a lot of time in bed or on the couch, and inevitably one or both of our cats was with him. Logan, a lovely, large part Maine Coon, was so faithful, so reliably there. They took comfort in each other, and Sabrina—our much older cat—frequently joined in. When Jim died, both cats were bereft. He spent the last two weeks of his life in the hospital, and the cats were noticeably confused; clearly they knew this was not an ordinary absence.

"Then about a year later, Logan died of a stroke at only 10. More heartbreak, more grief. An echo, if you will, of our grief, my daughter's and mine, at Jim's death. And a grief all its own, as well.

"My sister's experience was similar to mine but different. She and her husband, who died at a lamentably young age, had a dog, an Australian Shepherd. In his last weeks, John slept on a hospital bed in the living room—and Sydney slept beside him on that bed, cuddled close, keeping him company. This dog brought my sister comfort, too, both before John's death and afterward

"If you've experienced the loss of a long-time spouse, or someone close to you, you'll also understand that caring for the pets you shared (or for that matter, newly adopted pets) in as normal a way as possible can help you 'get through.'

"Jim and I had planned to get another dog after Willow, the last dog we had, died. And then he was diagnosed. A year-plus after his death, I finally fulfilled our plan. The dog's a rescue beagle who'd been substantially abused in her former 'home.' She has lasting injuries, and although I took on more than I'd expected, I adore this little girl (my 'bagel' as a young neighborhood boy called her). I feel our relationship—like all good people-animal relationships – is one of mutuality, of shared love, comfort and pleasure. And considering her previous life, Zelda's loving nature and her open friendliness is astonishing.

"Pets (which seems a rather condescending term to me) can support us in dealing with our grief. First, in the reassurance and company they consistently offer, as I've mentioned, and second, through the routine their care imposes on our lives—a responsibility in both practical and emotional ways.

"If the cat or dog (or rabbit or rodent!) was jointly yours and your spouse's or parent's or child's, there's also the matter of memory, which is both a consolation and a reminder that can bring sadness at first (for a while anyway), as well as a smile. With Sabrina, I feel that. She was with us for almost two decades (and is still with me).

"And when it comes to Zelda, I'm continually aware that Jim would have loved this little dog, too.

"Grief is complex. We all know that or at least sense it. And our relations with animals are also complex. (That's my opinion, but then I'm an editor, a reader and sometime writer, not a zoologist or psychologist.)

"I expect that some people see their relationships with a cat or dog as a simple, straightforward one. Feed. Walk. Change the litter. Throw the ball. Repeat. And even if that routine of caring is all there is, it still helps.

"But, please, let your animals be more to you! Take advantage of the opportunity they provide to be honest about your grief, to let them express theirs and to share with them all the special comforts we can."

Paula isn't the only person who told me how much a beloved animal helped during a time of grieving. Elaine VanEmon says, "I had a dog that forced me to get out of bed every morning. He would stand on top of me and bark 'til I finally crawled out of bed and took him out to potty. It was October and the temperature was brisk and woke me up fairly quickly. So then I was awake and would get ready for my day. Murphy (my dog) kept me from crawling into my bed and never getting out."

After reading what these women have shared, you might want to adopt an animal if you don't already own one.

It may take a while to reach, but at some point you will have to acknowledge that you have entered a new chapter in your life story. It will look different because a vital part of it is now gone, but it will still be your story and one worth continuing. If you're still here, there is still more to do, more to be.

This was brought home to me when we recently got to talking with a widower at a garage sale. He was selling his house and preparing to move to Oregon to a property with acreage and forest. He and his son were going to start a new life, buying a sawmill and going into the lumber business.

We don't want to lose precious memories but, while the past is a place we all love to visit, we can't remain there. I remember our pastor talking about a conversation he had with God after his wife died. "What do I do now?" he cried. "You live," came the answer. And he did. He kept on preaching, eventually met a lovely woman and remarried. This certainly didn't diminish the love he'd had for his wife, but he was still here and his story wasn't yet over. I suspect his first wife would very much approve of the choices he's made.

You may have married the love of your life and can't imagine anyone replacing him or her, and maybe no one ever will. But, as the saying goes, never say never. This world is filled with wonderful people. You might meet one of them. And sometimes remarrying benefits both parties, not only emotionally but also financially. If you are plagued with loneliness or if your spouse didn't leave you well provided for, remarrying might not be a bad idea. I think of my pal Roberta, who, at seventy decided she was tired of being a widow and met a very nice widower online on a site that catered to seniors. Together they enjoy traveling, going out to eat, and spending time with each other's family.

If death has visited you and taken away someone you loved let me assure you, you can survive the pain. In my own case and in the case of everyone I talked with, the sad times will still come long after the initial shock has worn off. But, as you move forward, so will some good times as well. Grieve, cope, and keep living. Know that there is no expiration date on moments of sadness. But know, too, that there is still a new chapter of your story to write.

1. Dr. Louis E. Lagrand, *Healing Grief, Finding Peace: 101Ways to Cope with the Death of Your Loved One*, (Source Books 2011).

8. HERE'S LOOKING AT YOU... STILL

I've been a mirror gazer since I was a teen. First it was inspecting my face for blackheads and zits. Then it was checking my make-up. Then, as I got older, it was checking out the wrinkle population, which has been growing steadily since I found my first one at age thirty-seven. Now, there's no gazing. Too scary.

Seeing all the procedures and skin cream products on the market, it's not hard to reach the conclusion that I'm not alone in how I feel about my aging reflection. I have friends who are getting face peels, face lifts, having those little dents filled in and paying for collagen injections in their lips, and I understand why they're doing it. For the same reason I dyed my hair starting with that first gray hair in my early thirties. Who wants to look like an old lady?

But really, in the long run, no matter what we do we will never look twenty again. And would you want to be twenty again? Most people I talk to answer that with a resounding no, probably because most of us did a lot of dumb things in our twenties. Who wants to repeat that?

This is not to say that you shouldn't have work done if you want to. My other half celebrated a landmark birthday by having the pouches under his eyes removed. If this is a burning need, I'm not going to stop you. But I'm leery of stretching out on the operating table and spending a fortune on a complicated procedure that could backfire. Remember Olivia Goldsmith, who wrote *The First Wives Club*? She died on the operating table having plastic surgery. You may be thinking, how often does that happen? My answer to that would have to be, "I don't know. But I don't want to wind up being the next fluke where something went wrong." *Remember Sheila Roberts? Yeah, she wanted an everything lift. Too bad she's no longer with us.*

Although I will confess, I recently yielded to temptation and indulged in a non-invasive treatment for my neck, thinking it would save me from being mistaken for a turkey come November. I have to say I think that was one of the dumbest things I've done in a long time. It hurt! A lot.

The experience didn't begin well. First of all, there was the paperwork to go over – pages of things that could go wrong. *You do understand this could happen, right? Initial here.*

"The chances are one in a million," the aesthetician at my dermatologist's office assured me as I began to hyperventilate.

One in a million. I'd be fine. Wouldn't I? I signed with a shaking hand and let her escort me to a treatment room to meet the machine that would transform me. It looked like a baby water heater. Once I was settled in a nice, comfy chair (with my head held in place by a padded brace) the aesthetician took from the magic machine what looked like a vacuum cleaner extension and hooked it on my neck. Then strapped it on.

There it sat, like a giant leech. Trying to crush my windpipe.

"It's crushing my windpipe," I informed her.

"Can you breathe?" she asked.

Well, yes. I obviously had enough breath to protest.

"Can you swallow?"

Sort of. "But it's crushing my windpipe!"

"It's really not," she assured me, making some final adjustments. "You'll be fine. Don't worry. I do this a lot and I've never lost a patient."

There was always a first time.

She turned on the vacuum, which really wasn't vacuuming anything. Instead it was freezing my fat cells. And trying to crush my windpipe.

After making sure all was well, she promised to be back to check on me, then left me in the chair with my head in the brace, pillows under the vacuum cleaner/leech, taking deep breaths to calm myself.

It was not a quick process. I had plenty of time for regrets. All the while I kept praying, "God, I'm so sorry I was vain. There are people starving in the world and I'm paying to have a giant ice leech hanging on my neck. I will never do this again. Ever!"

I plan to stick to that vow. Yes, I like my pretty new neck, and I now have less wrinkles so the procedure worked. And I suffered no ill-effects. But, like the Terminator in the old Arnold Schwarzenegger movie, those wrinkles will be back. So really, all I was doing was postponing the inevitable. I've decided I'm better off accepting who I am and where I am in life.

Having said all that, let me reiterate, if you feel the need to, as the saying goes, get some work done, I'm not going to stop you. I understand that it's important to feel good about ourselves. But if I start feeling the need, please lock me in my room.

No matter how hard I wind it, I won't be able to turn back the clock, so I'm determined to concentrate on looking polished and healthy and happy and leave it at that. I'll keep my vintage outside spruced up and put my energy into continuing to become a better version of myself. On the inside. Where the leeches can't get me.

As I'm writing this chapter, I happen to be reading Willie Nelson's autobiography. Over the years, Willie Nelson has collected a million wrinkles, and that scruffy beard and long, braided hair have become his trademarks. But does anyone care about those wrinkles and the fact that the hair is gray? He's Willie Nelson, for crying out loud, and his fans love him. As I examine Willie's face on the cover of that book I think, *Yep, he is sure old.* And then I think *Who cares? It's Willie.* It's not Willie's looks everyone loves, it's his talent, it's the songs he's written.

And how about the actress Diane Keaton? She's aging, but her fans haven't stopped going to movies she's in because she's getting old. They go because they love seeing her on screen and love the quirky characters she plays.

Cindy Joseph, the elegant senior fashion model who created the Boom cosmetic line says, "A woman's face tells an individual life story. Our beauty is born of self-knowledge, confidence and wisdom. Let's reveal and celebrate the beauty we've earned! Let's do it for ourselves and the young men and women in our society looking up to us for inspiration. You look fabulous as you are. It's your/our decision. Through example we have the power to change society's points of view about aging. You have vitality, joy and wisdom. Let the beauty you gained shine through."[1]

I need to recite that to myself every time I look in the mirror and am tempted to wish I looked thirty. Or forty. Heck, I'd settle for fifty. But how about I settle for the age I am?

Along those lines, fashion designer Diane Von Furstenberg says, "My face carries all my memories. Why would I erase them?"[2] Indeed!

Do you know who was voted sexiest man of the century in 1999? Sean Connery. He was fifty-nine at the time. Do you know who pops up regularly on Facebook as many women's heart-throb? Sam Elliot. As of this writing he's seventy-four.

Guys, you know what attracts us women? It's strength and confidence. And you can have that at sixty as well as at forty.

And ladies, not every old man is looking for a younger babe. As I write this I'm thinking of a woman I see regularly at our local Elks club. She's not a beauty by any means, but she's bubbly and sweet and knows how rock a dress. She never lacks for men to take her out dancing.

Think about your favorite older people in your life growing up, the ones who rooted for you, listened to your problems and applauded your successes, the people who shared their time with you and taught you how to do things like crochet and fish and bake cookies. Did you really spend much time thinking about their looks? Didn't you simply enjoy being with them? Do you think the people who care about you care any less because you're starting to show signs of having lived a long time? Hopefully, you answered that question with a resounding, "No."

I'm not advocating you go around looking like a slob or that you abandon shaving and washing. Crusty old guys who wear stained shirts and smell aren't exactly inspiring. And, unless you're in a movie portraying a bag lady, there's no need to dress in dowdy, ill-fitting clothes. No matter what our age or budget we can still look classy. (More on that in a bit!)

Let's take a moment and talk about some affordable ways we can all look like the fabulous seniors we are.

Beauty Products

Most of us spend a lot of money on face creams and moisturizers. This is hardly surprising since, as we get older, we lose the hormones that keep our skin oily. Some of those skin creams cost a fortune, which sure doesn't make them an option for people on a limited income. But never fear, you can still take care of your skin. Coconut oil does wonders for dry skin and is affordable. You can also use it on your hair and on your nails to keep them from cracking. Other natural oils such as olive oil are great as well. I'll often dab olive oil on my face for extra moisture. If you prefer to buy hand cream and body lotion, be sure to check the ingredients listed on the jar. Often you'll find the same ingredients listed on the label of a cheaper brand as the ones on the pricier version.

I love to listen to Dr. Jerry Mixon on the radio, and I remember on more than one occasion him sharing the mantra he was given as a doctor working with elderly patients: keep old skin oiled, wash when soiled. There it is in a nutshell, moisturize, moisturize, moisturize. Otherwise you'll end up with leg dandruff. Eew. Or plain, old itchy skin.

Your Smile

At a little beauty seminar I attended on our anniversary cruise the cosmetician asked us this question, "Who's the most beautiful woman in the world?"

Of course, I began to mentally tick off movie stars. Audrey Hepburn, Jacylyn Smith, Charlize Theron.

Our expert didn't drop a single name though. Instead, she said, "The woman with a beautiful smile."

Yes, a smile lights up the whole face, and that is something easily enhanced. For starters, simply whitening our teeth can make a difference. My dental assistant did inform me though that as we get older our teeth become less porous. So, if you've tried over the counter whitening strips without much luck, that's the reason why. You might have to try something stronger. Talk to your dentist and see what he or she can do for you. And be sure to brush your teeth after you drink tea or coffee because both are notorious for staining.

Ladies, get to your local cosmetician and pick out a lipstick that works with your skin color. Sometimes we need to adapt our make-up as we get older, tone things down just a little. What looks dramatic on a thirty-year old could appear clownlike on a seventy-year old. Guild the lily tastefully.

Clothes

You've probably heard the expression, clothes make the man.

Erasmus said this in the Middle Ages. Shakespeare said it. So did Mark Twain, and then added, "Naked people have little or no influence in society." There is something deep in our psyche that insists we respect people who dress well. Hence when our politicians are out stumping, they're in suits and power ties. When an organization throws a gala event, attendees are in tuxes and evening gowns. We look at a well-dressed man or woman and think, Success. We see a woman who dresses well as classy. And remember John T. Molloy and his *Dress For Success* books? Granted, styles have changed since that book came out and many of us are more casual now, even in the workplace, but most of us still, in some way or other, dress to impress.

Purchasing clothes at your local department store can get spendy, and if you're on a limited income that can be discouraging. But that doesn't mean you can't have a nice wardrobe. Consignment stores and thrift stores often offer a treasure trove of outfits for very little. I've picked up designer outfits and clothes with the store price tags still on them for peanuts. My favorite tale is the Tadashi blouse I found at Goodwill for ten dollars. Later I looked this brand up on line and about fell off my chair when I saw that similar blouses were going for a hundred and fifty dollars... on sale. I've found everything from evening gowns to bowling shirts for my husband. Great fun. I've also found all kinds of accessories at garage sales.

Of course, you can also buy at your favorite department store. Just wait until the sales start. Buy at the end of the season for the following year. Styles don't change that much in one season. Buy classics and update with your accessories.

Speaking of updating, ladies, let's remember to replace worn out bras. No one I know enjoys going bra shopping, but no one I know likes looking droopy and dumpy either. These days control top panties will also do wonders for our figures. If you'd like to look your best, a good foundation will make all the difference in how your clothes fit. So force yourself. Get a fitting and then splurge. And if you find a bra or panty you really like I'd encourage you to buy more than one. Many are the times I bought the perfect bra, only to find that style long gone when I went back to the store to get another.

When you do go on the hunt for clothes, take someone with you who will give you an unbiased opinion. I can always count on my best buddy Jan to tell me if a pair of pants or a top isn't flattering. If you're a man who's found himself suddenly single, enlist the help of a female friend or relative when picking out clothes.

And don't feel guilty about spending some money on looking good. You've worked hard all your life. It's okay to enjoy yourself a little now. We all have our own unique style. Find yours and rock it.

But remember, it will rock better if you're keeping in good physical shape. Lose that tummy fat. Not only will you look better without it, you'll decrease the odds of cancer. For some reason, that fat around our middles makes a great host for cancer cells.[3]

Also, don't be afraid to change or fine tune your style. Maybe you've reached the point where you're tired of dying your hair. It's okay to go gray. Look how gorgeous Glenn Close looks with her gray hair. And Jamie Lee Curtis. And how about Richard Gere? That man looks great in gray.

If you're a guy and your hair is disappearing, you have my permission to shave your head. You've probably heard the saying, "God only made so many perfect heads. The rest He covered with hair." There you have it. If you've got a "perfect" head (as in the hair is going) don't be ashamed to show it off. Think of Yul Brynner and Dwayne Johnson, "the Rock." As one of my girlfriends recently said, bald beats a comb over any day.

Baldness in women can be another matter. It's very hard on us ladies when our hair starts to thin. While this is a culture that acknowledges male pattern baldness, it's not so kind to women who find their hair thinning. And many of us do. I know mine certainly isn't what it was before chemo.

If your hair is thin you might consider having your hormones tested. I recently learned from a friend that too much testosterone in women as we age can leave us with extra chin hairs and not enough hair on the top of our heads. She had hers tested and the doctors gave her a choice. She could either up her estrogen (which came with its own set of risks) or suppress her testosterone. The medication for that didn't carry the same risky side effects, so she chose the magic testosterone-reducing pill. I've got to say, her hair looks great. Little Sheila is going to be asking her doctor about this at her next post-cancer check-up. You might want to consult your doctor as well.

Or you could invest in a good wig. One of my buddies has done that, joking that the only thing on her which got slim was her hair. If, like her, you're feeling the need to cover up you can find all manner of high-quality wigs on line or in a specialty shop. When I was going through my chemo-bald phase my husband and I found a shop in Seattle that specialized in women's wigs. It was good to be able to try on several to see which one looked the best.

A quick aside here. If you are undergoing chemo, your insurance company may pick up the tab for a wig (hair prosthesis) if your oncologist writes you a prescription. If your insurance won't cover this cost, organizations such as Wigs and Wishes and Lolly's Locks provide free wigs for cancer victims. You can find both these organizations on line.

Hearing Aids

You may be wondering why on earth I'm talking about hearing aids in a chapter on looking our best. I'm bringing up this subject because many of us are leery of getting them, even when we need them. We worry that people will see them and think we're going deaf. To many they are stigmatizing.

Well, I have news for you. If you're going deaf you need them.

Due to years spent playing in bands, my hearing had deteriorated. Finally, after a long flight I wound up with such a buzzing in my ear I was sure I had an auditory aura from a migraine. But the headache never showed, and in spite of all the medicine I took that noise refused to go away. I finally went to a specialist and learned that I had significant hearing loss. Which would explain my often asking, "What?" after someone spoke to me. I fought the idea of hearing aids. To me that was the ultimate sign that I am – shudder – old. It took a lot of self-lecturing for me to go from needing hearing aids to getting hearing aids. What finally did it was reminding myself that I'd worn glasses and contact lenses for years so I could see better. There really was no difference in getting something to help me hear better than there was in getting something to help me see better. So I made the leap. And, I'm happy to say that I do, indeed, hear better.

Today's hearing aids are so small the average person never notices them. Mine match my hair color and are hidden under my hair. They're the best accessory I've ever purchased. That might turn out to be the case for you as well.

Sleep

It's not only good for our health, it's also good for our looks. As we get older our skin loses its elasticity and that thin skin under our eyes can get darker. A poor night's sleep only makes it worse. The same is true for those smile lines (nasolabial folds) that run from each side of the nose to the corners of the mouth. The Thanksgiving we stayed overnight with one of my brothers and sisters-in-law and slept in really comfy bed I made an amazing discovery. Those smile lines, which had been looking like the Grand Canyon disappeared over night! I took a double take when I looked in the mirror the next morning, sure that I was hallucinating. Or that my sister-in-law had bought water taken from the Fountain of Youth. But no, I wasn't hallucinating and we'd drunk no magic potion. I'd simply slept really well.

Good Food

Here's another help for those dark circles under our eyes (and other parts of our body as well): leafy green vegetables. Spinach, kale, and broccoli contain vitamin K, which helps with blood coagulation and circulation. Poor circulation can exacerbate those pesky dark circles, so do your part to fight them and veggie up. (Unless you're on certain blood thinners. Then take it easy and don't overload on the spinach and kale.) If you enjoy the goodies found in the popular Mediterranean Diet (olive oil, tomatoes, leafy greens, and fruit) you'll be taking in antioxidants that help block the chemical reactions that lead to sun damage. Fresh produce neutralizes those free radicals that contribute to wrinkles, brown spots and other signs of aging. [4]

It can seem so vain to focus on how we look. Still, I think looking our best is important because when we look good we feel good. Taking care of our bodies is rather like taking care of anything we've been given, whether it's a house, a car or a new stove. We show our appreciation for what we have by treating it well. So let's treat ourselves well.

Let's also remember that, while packaging is pretty, it's still what's inside that counts. The wrinkles are going to come and things are going to sag. But if we keep our souls beautiful those who love us won't give the wrinkles even a passing thought, especially when they're admiring our great suit or hot shoes.

1. I got permission from Cindy's organization to quote her and was saddened recently to see that she lost her battle with cancer.

2. Diane von Furstenberg, *The Woman I Wanted to Be*, (Simon and Schuster, 2014), p. 121.
3. Nbcnews.com: *Belly Fat Increases Risk of Breast Cancer Despite Normal BMI, Study Finds*, Copyright 2019.

HTTPS://WWW.NBCNEWS.COM/HEALTH/WOMENS-HEALTH/BELLY-FAT-INCREASES-RISK-BREAST-CANCER-DESPITE-NORMAL-BMI-STUDY-N951246

1. Forbes.com: *The Best Diets for Your Skin*, Copyright 2019.

https://www.health.com/beauty/the-best-diets-for-your-skin?slide=104265#104265

9. NOT LIMITED BY A LIMITED INCOME

Those retirement years can sneak up on us. Sometimes they sneak up and say, "Boo!"

If you're getting ready to retire, let me share some good advice from finance guru Suze Orman.[1] She recommends you divide your spending into two buckets: needs and wants. Your needs are, obviously your essential monthly bills – housing insurance, food, utilities, taxes, gas and medical expenses. You'll add up your income including Social Security Benefits and any pension, required minimum distributions taken from your 401 (k) and IRA accounts. Needs will get paid out of those. Your wants, the fun stuff in that second bucket, will come out of the savings you have leftover. Or any extra money you may happen to earn. (More on that later.)

Here's hoping you planned well for your gold-plated years and there is plenty of money for both the needs and the wants. Suze does caution that many people overspend early in retirement and run short of cash later, so make sure you're setting aside enough money for needs, making allowance for inflation and unexpected financial challenges.

If you're retired and feeling the financial pinch, never fear. I have some suggestions for ways you can still enjoy life, even if you're enjoying it on less money than you'd like.

Enhancing Your Income

First, let's talk about ways you might be able to get a little more money.

Reverse Mortgage

The HECM (home equity conversion mortgage) is, at the time of this writing, available to seniors sixty-two and older, and is a new wrinkle on going into debt. Your house is free and clear? Great! Give it back to the bank.

Okay, my bias is showing and I'm only including this because I'm sure someone reading this book may be considering a reverse mortgage as an option. I personally think this is a terrible idea because after you're dead someone else has to pay off your debt by selling the house, probably your children. For many of us, the most valuable asset we have to leave our heirs is our home. Taking out a reverse mortgage will impact how much you're able to leave. In other words, the kids will only get the equity that wasn't borrowed against.

Now, if you don't happen to be speaking to your children, then great. That'll teach the little beasts. But if you're wanting to pass on something to help the next generation financially this is a sure way to put a spike in that wheel because the loan will have to be repaid once your house is sold. If you move, the loan also needs to get paid back, just as if you still carried a mortgage on your house. So there go your profits. With a reverse mortgage you're not making payments and gaining equity, you're taking payments from your equity.

Here's another thought. Many of us think of our house as a safety net, something we can sell in case we need special care further down the road. A reverse mortgage will chew up a considerable amount of that money.

There are, however, many who would still argue for getting a reverse mortgage. If you are about to run out of money, this may be your only option.

Here are some facts for you that I picked up courtesy of bankrate.com. This mortgage loan program enables seniors to withdraw some of the equity on their home if they need money. The loans come with fees, starting with an origination fee that ranges from $2,500 to $6,000. It doesn't require monthly mortgage payments but you do have to pay your homeowners insurance, and taxes, and maintain your home. A reverse mortgage can delay your having to pay taxes when you begin drawing down on your 401(k) plan, thus delaying the associated taxes. Obviously, this is complicated, and you'd be well advised to consult an expert in this field who can explain all this to you in more detail if you're considering it.

I do understand the frustration of having too much month at the end of the money. In the early years of my marriage we lived on a budget tighter than support hose. (Although we still managed to have fun – something I talk about in more detail in my book *How to Live Large on a Small Budget*.) Lean periods are part of life and at some point, most of us land in that uncomfortable place.

Many of us land there at a time in life when it can be a challenge to go out and get more money. According to the Economic Policy Institute, retirement wealth has not grown fast enough to keep pace with an aging population and other changes.[2]

If you happen to have gotten caught in the uh-oh, we-don't-have-enough-money trap, then this might be an option for you. If you're cash strapped and barely getting by this may be your only option. Also, you can use a reverse mortgage to settle your existing mortgage debt or home equity line of credit. Just remember, somebody, probably your heirs, will be paying this off at some point.

According to the article on bankrate that I quoted earlier, reverse mortgage borrowers are required to undergo counseling with an independent third-party HECM counselor, who will go over all the features with them, discuss different loan product options and the costs and even discuss your expenses and budget. A very good idea. Even what seems like the easiest fix can have its side effects. Best to be aware of them before you commit.

And with that, I want to circle back one more time to my soap box. According to my favorite financial guru, Dave Ramsey, reverse mortgages are loaded with extra costs. He cautions that you could find yourself in trouble as those costs mount up.[3] So, again, caveat emptor. Let the buyer beware. Do what you gotta do, but do your research.

Downsizing

Instead of a reverse mortgage you might want to consider downsizing. If your house is free and clear but too big and too much work, why not move to something smaller in size and cost? You will, most likely, come out ahead after fees and capital gains taxes, and be left with some extra money to invest.

Collectibles

Do you have some valuable collectibles? Perhaps it's time to sell off some of them. Got some old Star Wars action figures? Pez dispensers? How about old comic books? The 1938 Action Comic Book where the world first met Superman went for 3.2 million on Ebay.[4] First editions, especially if they're signed, can bring in money to invest or live on. So can some of those toys you or your kids played with. Do an online search (or enlist the help of a grandchild – they're all internet savvy!) and see what some of that stuff you have kicking around is worth. Selling collectibles can be a profitable first step in downsizing.

Recently, my other half and I went to our local coin store and sold some old gold jewelry that was broken or never worn. We came away with a tidy sum.

Perhaps you have some art that you once loved that doesn't do it for you anymore. Or a coin collection. Valuable baseball cards. These are all the types of things we usually want to save to pass on to family members. But, if the need arrives, they can also be a source of revenue.

Ebay

You might want to sell some treasures on eBay or start your own eBay store. I recently saw a porcelain Kewpie doll like the one my mother-in-law gave me on that site selling for a hundred bucks. (Don't worry, Mom. I'm not going to sell it!) That brings us back to the hidden treasures, doesn't it? Once in a while you might find some great goodies at garage sales and, once in a while, at your local thrift store, that you can turn around and sell. When we were putting our son through college and the writing profits were skimpy this was one of many ways I earned tuition money. I loved the thrill of the hunt and enjoyed watching as the bids on my offerings grew. You might also.

Part-time Work

We talked in an earlier chapter about starting your own business. Even if you don't want to work that long and that hard, there are things you can do part-time to bring in extra income. Tutoring, substitute teaching, greeting at Walmart, selling cosmetics, offering handyman services, giving art or piano lessons, taking pictures at weddings – these are all ways we can supplement our retirement income. If you love to work with wood or paint flowers on glassware or are clever and crafty, you can participate in craft fairs.

If none of those ideas appeal, how about pet sitting or house sitting? This can be a great way to both earn some extra income and get to stay in some very nice homes. We have some pals near our beach digs who have a pet sitter more than willing to help them out as she not only gets to play with their dogs, she also gets a mini-vacation in a lovely beach home. And then, there's plain old house-sitting. Get paid to watch someone else's TV!

You might want to try participating in what's referred to as the sharing economy – driving for Uber, making that downstairs bed and bath available on Airbnb or using TaskRabbit to offer your skills.

Who knows what opportunities are waiting for you? A few phone calls, a post in your community's Facebook page or the local paper and you could be in business.

And, speaking of business and working, according to RetirementJobs.com[5]. once you are over your full retirement age your earnings will have no impact on your social security. (In other words, Uncle Sam can't say, "Hey, you earned more money than I allowed you. Now give some of it back.") Stop by your local Social Security branch and discuss this with someone to see what that age is for you. (We actually double-checked this as I had nightmares about getting in a mess and having to pay back taxes. For your own peace of mind I encourage you to do the same.

Living Better on Less

Now that we've enhanced your income, let's talk about ways to control your budget without limiting your fun. There are so many ways we can get what we want and enrich our lives without breaking our piggy banks. Here are a few suggestions.

. . .

Bartering

Perhaps you don't have the energy or inclination to commit to a steady job even if it is part-time. You can still make your skills work for you. A little old-fashioned bartering will get you all kinds of things. Know how to cut hair? How about offering haircuts in exchange for car maintenance? Or trading lawn service for baked goodies and homemade jam or canned goods? Home-cooked meals in exchange for some handyman help? Or maybe you want to give those piano lessons in exchange for a weekend at someone's summer cabin or time share. Be willing to wheel and deal.

I've seen several friends who dealt themselves into staying in some scenic parks by offering their services as hosts (or visitor center docents) in exchange for a place to park their travel trailer for free and enjoy outdoor adventure. My friend Doreen and her husband are doing this and having a wonderful time. Their job entails cleaning campsites after people depart, answering questions as needed, selling firewood (depending on the park), and posting reservations tags as needed. In return for this light work they receive a full hook-up campsite and several hours off each work day. Current rate for a campsite in my state of Washington is forty to forty-five dollars a night. Over time, that's a nice saving. Even better than the savings, according to Doreen, is the fact that this allows them to see places they might not go if it were simply for a night. The people they've met, some of whom have become friends, are a bonus. If you love the outdoors and want to see more of the U.S.A. this could be worth looking into.

Investigate ushering at your local community theater. I have several friends who do this, both at the charming vintage theater in our town and in nearby Seattle. In exchange for helping people find their seats they can see shows for free. At the price of theater tickets, that's a great deal.

We've all heard the old saying that one man's junk is another man's treasure. Maybe it's time to do some treasure swapping.

The women in my old neighborhood loved doing this. We would gather two or three times a year and swap goodies. It started with a jewelry swap at my house. Everyone brought old costume jewelry she never wore anymore and we traded. It was so much fun we continued the tradition, swapping everything from clothes to household items. My girlfriends at the beach do this once a year, gathering for an annual swap party. Great fun to trade stuff back and forth.

Sharing

Remember Mama always telling you to share? That advice can pay off big if you're on a limited income. While we can't all afford to run out and buy a boat, a camper, a time share or a cabin on the lake, we might be able to access those big-ticket items by going in together with family members or friends.

Obviously, getting along well is a prerequisite. And, no matter how well you get along and how much you love each other, you need to get things in writing before investing. Know ahead of time all the costs and who will be responsible for what. Will everything be split down the middle or will it be sixty-forty with the family owning the lion's share of the big toy getting to use it the most or will it be fifty-fifty? Who will use it when? Will you use it together? (Hopefully, the answer to that is yes.) Will you have an option for one of you to buy out the other when someone wants out or will you both have to sell? And if you do, how will the profits be split? Putting those details in writing beforehand will save you misunderstandings and hard feelings further down the road if and when circumstances change. (And, life being what it is, they will.)

You can share more than cabins and campers. Why not share that riding lawn mower or chain saw with your neighbor? My girlfriend at the beach and I have gone in together on crabbing supplies, which makes perfect sense as we plan to catch many crabs together. Never mind that our first outing was like an episode of *I Love Lucy*. We broke our little crab trap and about drowned ourselves wading around in the surf. But we had fun and have high hopes for future success. We'll also be investing in more equipment.

That same neighbor and her husband have allowed us, the part-timers, to add our garbage and recycle items to their cans. I give her a small amount of money (and a new novel whenever one comes out) and we piggy back onto them, which saves us from having to pay for a garbage service we wouldn't use much of the year.

Taking trips together can be both fun and affordable. How about renting a camper with a sibling or another couple and taking a road trip? A good way to see the country and at half the price. Or perhaps simply go somewhere local. I take a yearly trip with my pals, the Game Girls, each year to a different location within a few hours' drive of our homes and this is very affordable fun as we all share the expense of the gas and split the cost of a room. Great good times on a budget. Last year we stayed at the beautiful Quinault Lodge on Washington's Olympic Peninsula. The scenery was breathtaking and the time with friends priceless.

My family has done something similar in the past, renting a large house for the weekend and bringing our own food to cook. This can be a fun memory maker and easy on the budget. Three couples going in together to stay at a vacation on the beach versus one couple – this is the kind of math even those of us who are math challenged can do.

Speaking of traveling, if you enjoy travel and happen to speak a foreign language fluently, you can earn yourself a free trip by turning yourself into a tour guide and taking a small group to some of your favorite places in a foreign country. My husband did this several times earlier in our marriage. He's fluent in German and lived much of his life in Germany, so was able to make his small tours personal and interesting, introducing his travelers to both historical sights and local people. Of course, you have to like to plan trips, have an eye for detail and be well insured if you plan to do something like this. And you have to have good people skills because things don't always go as planned.

Contests

Yes, I know. What are the chances of winning something? Better than if you don't enter, I can tell you that. Radio stations often have contests running where you can win money or concert tickets, on-line reader blogs and sites such as Goodreads all offer book giveaways, and most authors, such as myself, usually have contests going on their websites and/or Facebook pages. Throughout the year I've given away everything from saltwater taffy to Christmas ornaments.

It's not always about the size of your winnings. Sometimes it's simply fun to win. Who doesn't like getting a goody in the mail? I remember being thrilled the time I won a free Helen Reddy album from my local radio station. (Boy, did I just date myself!) My husband once answered a trivia question correctly and won us tickets to a Ryan Adams concert. Fun times.

Blogging

Are you a big reader? Do you love sharing your thoughts? Perhaps it's time to start blogging. Many bloggers review books which gives them the double benefit of talking books with other readers and, if they have a following, scoring free books from publishers or self-published authors who are wanting the exposure for their latest creative output. You get a free book and review it and the writer gets exposure. A win-win for all.

. . .

Foraging

This is one of my favorite activities. In the summer I love to pick berries and fill up my freezer for winter. Smoothies, homemade blackberry pie and jam – oh, yes. In the fall we've spent many happy afternoons wandering around the woods with friends, hunting mushrooms. Remember how much fun you had as a child looking for Easter Eggs? Well, this is like Easter Egg hunting for grown-ups. So much fun. And at the end of the day you have 'shrooms for omelets, spaghetti sauce and cream of mushroom soup. In our area huckleberries ripen in the late summer and fall and yes, my friends and I scrounge those as well. Fishing, crabbing, shrimping, clam digging, hunting – if you live in an area where you can do these things, go for it. Yes, for some of this you need a license, but if you go out often enough that license will more than pay for itself. Thank God that so far nobody is making me pay for the privilege of picking berries!

Bargain Hunting

At this point in life there's little we need, but if you do find yourself needing anything from new lawn care equipment to candles, think outside the big box store. The best bargains to be found are in what's often referred to as the underground economy. Online buy and swap sites and garage sales are all treasure troves and a real boon to anyone on a limited income. Hitting garage sales has become a popular American pastime, right up there with baseball, and going with friends turns the whole thing into a party. Half the furnishings in our beach home I picked up at garage sales. Oh, the finds we've found over the years, everything from beds to wine glasses and espresso machines. So much fun and such a money saver. I'm convinced that if you wait long enough you can get anything you need or want at a garage sale.

. . .

Life Enriching Activities

Want to feel good about yourself? Stop thinking about yourself. Get out there and do something for others. You might even be able to put your passion to use. When I was getting my chemo treatments I enjoyed wearing scarves and hats knitted by many wonderful women. My pal Doreen, who I mentioned earlier, loves to crochet, and before she hit the road with her husband, she was in a club that met on a regular basis and made blankets to give to people who were going through hard times. The women not only indulged their passion for creating, they also passed on comfort to people going through trying times.

If you have a gift for organizing your local school or church would probably love to have your help. If you're a talker, consider doing some phoning for your political party or favorite charitable cause when they're raising funds.

Your Senior Center

Chances are your local senior center might offer activities that interest you. The one near me offers activities for everyone that range from line dancing, ping pong and pool to luncheons and excursions.

Some centers charge a modest yearly membership fee. Others are free to use and will charge for meals or classes. Check out the one nearest you and see what it has to offer.

Park and Rec

Your local park department will also offer any number of classes that may interest you. And if you don't want to take a class you may want to look into teaching one. (Another fun way to earn a little extra spending money.)

. . .

Clubs

It costs to join some clubs. For others the biggest cost will be your time. Book clubs are a great way to connect and many local libraries have book kits – boxes with several copies of a certain book that clubs can check out. If you don't have one going in your neighborhood or circle of friends check with your local library as they usually sponsor several clubs. You can find a club for almost anything, from chess or bridge to gardening, and they are a great way to build your social life by connecting with people who share your interests. (Of course, in addition to books and clubs, your local library offers all kinds of free entertainment: books, book readings, lectures, CDs and DVDs.)

Informal get-togethers can also be fun. How about gathering with some friends to ... play guitars and sing old rock and roll songs (my husband's favorite activity), play Bunco or board games, drive around in old cars, watch a chick flick or a fight or football game. We've gathered with friends many times to experiment in the kitchen, making a gourmet meal and splitting the cost of ingredients. Karen Oram-Proudfoot has her Ladies That Lash Club, a group of friends who get together to share beauty products, ideas, and morale boosting. (Karen, if I lived by you I'd so be joining that club!)

Living well isn't so much about what we make as it is about what we do. So don't let anyone tell you that a small income equals a small life. T'aint so.

1. Suze Orman, *The New Rules of Retirement, AARP Magazine*, August/September 2018.
2. Epi.org: Monique Morrissey, *The State of American Retirement: How 401(k)s Have Failed most American workers,* Economic Policy Institute, March 3, 2016.

HTTPS://WWW.EPI.ORG

1. Daveramsey.com: *The Reverse Mortgage: What Is It and How Does It Work?* Copyright 2019.

https://www.daveramsey.com/blog/how-reverse-mortgages-work

1. Goodhousekeeping.com: *The 40 Most Valuable Toys from Your Childhood*, Copyright 2019.

https://www.goodhousekeeping.com/childrens-products/toy-reviews/g3302/most-valuable-toys-from-childhood/?slide=7

1. RetirementJobs.com: *Will My Retirement Job Affect Social Security?*, Copyright 2019.

https://retirementjobs.com/career-advice/working-and-collecting-social-security/

10. BOOMER BEWARE

We all like to think we are much too smart to get taken in by crooks and con artists, but you never know. These people are clever, and the fact that the FBI has a web page dedicated to fraud against seniors proves that some of us are getting ripped off. Let's talk a little bit about what's out there and why it often comes looking for us.

According to the F.B.I.[1], we older and wiser types make good targets for several reasons. Many of us own our own home, have good credit and may even have some money in savings. We're walking piggy banks, waiting to be cracked open. Those of us who grew up in the forties or fifties were raised to be polite and trusting so we have a harder time saying no or hanging up on someone. For any number of reasons (including plain old embarrassment) we're less likely to report fraud. And sometimes we don't remember enough to provide all the necessary details to take down the crook.

It appears that women over the age of sixty make especially good targets for people selling products or services over the phone. Telemarketing scams often involve offers of free prizes, low-cost vitamins and health care and cheap vacations (and why would we go for the latter when we can use Groupon?)

So, what kind of scams should we be watching for?

Calls from Fake Government Officials

Scammers will call claiming to be from the County Clerk's office, saying they've been attempting to contact you. They might even cite a court case. Of course, because you haven't responded to these fake attempts you are now being fined. Pay up. Yes, the courthouse will happily take your credit card number.

Another big one is getting a call from someone official sounding claiming to have a warrant out for your arrest. You must make immediate payment if you want to stay out of jail. But, lucky you, you can pay the fine using a reloadable debit card or gift card.

You may also get a call from your local sheriff's office, informing you that you have unpaid parking tickets that you need to pay now. Or else.

Another big one is tax debts. Who doesn't walk in fear of the IRS? So when you get a call demanding you pay your tax debt – wait, what tax debt? – immediately. It's easy to go into panic mode and pay up in any way that official person tells you. This one is the most pervasive impersonation fraud in IRS history.

Grandparent Scams

In this con game the weasels phone grandparents with phony claims that a grandchild is in trouble and needs help paying a hospital bill or getting released from jail. Your grandchild may even have been overseas and gotten in trouble. Imagine that. Nobody told you little Junior was in Dubai, peddling drugs.

Sweetheart Scams

This one is as old as the hills, but it still works, especially on those of us who are lonely. Widows and widowers, people who are divorced – no matter what our gender, we're all equally vulnerable. According to an F.B.I. audio podcast I recently checked out the average financial loss from these schemes is between fifteen and twenty thousand dollars.[2] These days our technology and online dating sites make it easy for a scammer to bilk someone who is lonely and looking for love.

Of course, all starts out well, with pictures and interests shared. Often those pictures look nothing like the person with whom you're connecting, but that's all part of the illusion, just like those common interests. Of course, this person will seem wonderful and caring and you'll feel like you struck romance gold. As I write this I think of one friend who found someone who appeared to be the perfect man. He was in a high-powered job, working overseas. Very glam. But, as usually happens with these budding romances, there came a point when, although he really wanted to get back to the states to see her, he needed money because something horrible had happened. (Hint, hint.) Thank God my friend was smart enough not to send him any! By the way, once he realized he wasn't going to get any money he vanished.

Usually, these scammers are outside the country, so there's no way to catch and punish them. The money lost is rarely recovered.

Roofing Scams

According to one reputable roofing firm's site, scammers often seek out neighborhoods with a high percentage of seniors.[3] So, what do you need to look out for?

Storm chasers, for one. These people will often show up after a storm, looking for damaged roofs. They'll knock on your door, saying they just repaired a roof a few houses down and have extra material left over and have they got a deal for you. No, they don't.

It's a scam. They'll do poor work and then get out of town. To avoid this, check anyone out with the Better Business Bureau. Ask for local references and insurance information. Better yet, just tell them to blow away and go with someone local who is a part of your community.

Low ball bidders are not always your friend either. They may start out giving you lower estimates than any other roofer and then keep raising the price as you go along due to "unforeseen circumstances."

Then there are those eagle-eyed roofers who will spot imaginary roof damage on your house. Of course, they'll use jargon you can't understand. They may even sneak and do some of the damage themselves while "inspecting" your roof.

In addition to unscrupulous roofers, also watch out for crooks who try to pass off flying ants as termites and guys who happen to have leftover driveway sealant from (you guessed it) a job they just finished around the corner.

The Funeral Scam

This is a new one I've been seeing lately. Maybe you have, too. It would appear there are many kids and teens now dying and there is an urgent need for money to bury them. So, of course their friends all make signs on bits of cardboard that may read *R.I.P. Johnny*[4], *Funeral Donations Needed, Money Needed to Bury Ten-Year-Old George*. You'll find them alongside the street, with large plastic bottles needing to be filled with your hard-earned dollars. Even though this looks like a heartbreaking scenario (and it's meant to), there are better, legit ways to help a family in need after a death. If you want to help, get the name and address of the deceased, then do some internet sleuthing. I'm betting you won't find anything. If, however, you do, you'll probably find a fund has been set up for this individual either at a local financial institution or through GoFundMe, a legitimate donation site.

. . .

Identity Theft

This is on the rise, affecting more than eleven million people.[5] How does it happen? Any number of ways. Hacking, for one. We've all seen stories in the news about large chains getting hit, but hackers can find your information other ways as well, such as stealing your wallet or going through your garbage, looking for bank statements, pre-approved credit card offers or tax information. And, thanks to technology, clever thieves can easily lure in the unsuspecting.

Ever hear of Phishing? A phisher will create a webpage designed to look like the website of a bank or other financial institution. They'll send out email messages with a request that you take action. The email will have a link in it to – wait for it – their webpage. Once you've clicked on the link and entered your account number, thinking it's your bank, they've got you.

Then there's skimming, a practice that can be done with a scanning device that can be either hand held or strapped to an ankle. If an identity thief such as a clerk or waiter runs your credit card through his or her scanner you've got trouble. Ah, the joys of modern technology.

Scams Abroad

As many of us are enjoying travel at this time of our lives let me just take a moment to address a few popular scams you might encounter while traveling. One popular method of bilking tourists is the Petition Scam. Someone approaches you with a petition to sign (often the petitioner pretends to be deaf). Saying, "Sorry, I'm not from around here," will not get you off the hook. Because that has nothing to do with anything. The goal is to either get you to stand still and argue so your pocket can be picked or to sign your name and therefore commit yourself to forking over some money to the cause. Once you sign the petition, the petitioner then demands cash for whatever cause they were supposedly representing. We were hit twice by petitioners while at the Louvre, waiting for the museum to open and these women were aggressive, walking alongside and far from willing to take no for an answer. A very firm no finally sent each one on their way. Funny, how that deaf woman's hearing quickly improved!

Another popular scam a relative shared with me is the kind-hearted gift scam. This will involve someone making a cute little bracelet and putting it on your wrist as a gift. Except once it's on your wrist the giver would like a gift also: money. This, I learned from my niece, is also done using flowers. You're strolling the piazza, enjoying the romance of it all and a sweet little old man or lady will come up and give wifey a flower. A flower for the lady. Isn't that sweet? Then he'll turn to the gentleman and ask him to pay for the flower. If you're feeling generous, I guess you can overpay for a single flower. If not, give the flower back and walk away. (Which is exactly what my niece and her husband did.)

Pickpockets abound in Europe and I'm sure, if you're a traveler, you've been cautioned to keep your wallet hidden and your purse close to you. I would also encourage you to be aware of your surroundings, especially if you are hauling carry-on luggage behind you. How do I know this? Personal experience.

We had purchased tickets and gotten on the train leaving Paris, intending to spend the night at the airport before flying home. Lo and behold, three men had spotted us buying our tickets, seen my husband reaching into his man purse for his charge card, and then followed us onto the train. They had a system. The first man, who'd gotten on ahead of my husband, was the Distractor. My husband got on the train, which was relatively crowded and bustling, and the man grabbed his carry-on and began shaking it, talking in rapid-fire French. Clueless me, standing by, thought my husband had bumped him with it and now the irritated man was explaining train protocol. In fact, I thought he was trying to explain that there was a rack on the train for luggage. There wasn't. What was I thinking? Meanwhile, as he was creating a commotion, Man Number two, was edging my husband away from me, herding him like a two-legged sheep dog. And what was Man Number Three doing? Reaching his hand into my husband's bag. Happily, my husband saw his greedy little paw and slapped it away. The jig was up and the Distractor asked in French, "Are we good?" Then decided we were and, without waiting for an answer, he and his cohorts dashed off the train right as the doors were closing.

I didn't have a clue what had happened until we found seats and my husband related his adventure. And, I have to admit, I was shocked at how oblivious I'd been to what was going on.

A man two seats down said, "You know what they were trying to do. They were trying to rob you."

Yes, we did. And we were grateful that they didn't succeed.

The man shook his head in disgust and assured us that "This isn't France."

We had to agree. With the exception of the petitioners and our trio of sneaky thieves, everyone we'd met had been kind and helpful.

But there will always be that element, people who prefer to hardly work rather than work hard, people who would rather cheat their way to an extra buck, people who would rather take your money than earn their own. And chances are that at some point you'll meet one (or more) of them.

Here's my advice after our adventure:

Keep your money well out of sight – hide your wallet, stuff that credit card in your bra – and don't flash your wealth. Leave your best bling at home.

Also be aware that even without your bling, thieves will assume that since you're a foreigner that you're rich. After all, you're traveling, right? So try not to look like a foreigner. Dress nicely and find some walking shoes that aren't tennis shoes. Don't simply gawk and take pictures, buy some of that local produce. And don't start a love affair with the Millennials' favorite toy, the selfie stick. You and yourselfie will stick out like a narcissistic sore thumb.

Getting around a country with the locals is great fun, but to and from the airport opt for a cab or Uber rather than walk to your home away from home dragging your luggage behind you (which is the equivalent of wearing a sign on your back that says, "Rob me.")

If you don't speak a country's language fluently, consider visiting it in a group with a knowledgeable tour guide. And try to at least learn a few basic words in that country's language. (It may not save you from getting robbed but it will make the natives a lot more sympathetic to your cause.)

Read up on scams and things to beware of before you leave town. Forewarned is forearmed. There are a number of travel sites on line where you can learn about other popular scams, and if you're going to be traveling, I'd encourage you to do so.

Sometimes we're in danger from people we should be able to trust. None of us like to think a beloved son or daughter or grandchild would cheat us out of our hard-earned money, but it can happen. Adult children can gain access to credit and ATM cards and charge things without asking our permission. They can forge checks. They can get dependent parents to sign a deed, will, contract, or power of attorney through deception, coercion, or undue influence.

Often we get sucked into these situations because we are simply trying to help. We take in an adult child who's struggling financially or a grandchild who's had problems and the person we're trying to help brings those problems into our homes.

Those of us who don't have family can be equally vulnerable, forming close relationships with caregivers who, eventually take advantage of us. Where does it all end?

Or, more to the point, how can we avoid it beginning in the first place? Let's talk about ways we can protect ourselves.

Put on Your Armor

Shred or burn documents and don't leave things out in the open where people can see them. This is especially true if you have in-home caregivers or people coming in to clean. Have a file box with a lock for your important papers and keep it locked. Also, keep your most valuable jewelry in a safe. Better yet, get a safety deposit box at your local bank and store your most valuable items and important papers there.

Hire an identity theft protection service or get identity theft insurance. If you suspect someone has stolen or gotten ahold of your social security number, put a security freeze on your credit file with the three credit bureaus (Equifax, Experian and TransUnion).

Don't answer the phone when you see a number you don't recognize. If it's someone you need to talk to that person will leave a message.

Don't panic if you receive an alarming phone message, and don't call back until you've done some investigating. Chances are you're not about to go to jail and the sheriff won't be knocking on your door and no one in your family is being held for ransom in Transbanabuck. Call your bank, the courthouse, whoever and make sure the person who just called you really is who he said he was.

Don't provide your financial information to anyone who calls you. This especially applies to calls you might get from someone claiming to be from the customer service or fraud department of your bank or credit card company. Whatever has "happened," whatever that person is "looking into," you can also look into on your own. End the conversation and call the bank or credit card company yourself (and don't use the number the caller gave you.)

Also, the IRS does not call people about their taxes. It sends a letter. So don't panic when you get a call from "the tax man."

If you pick up the phone and, lo and behold, there is someone selling you something fabulous, be on the watch for the following phrases:

"You have to act now. This offer will expire soon."

"Congratulations, you've won a ________. You'll just need to pay for postage and handling."

"You must send money."

"You must give a credit card or bank account number or have a check picked up by courier." (Give my bank account number? Seriously?)

"There's no need for references. This is a solid company."

If you hear these from a salesman, do not pass Go, do not lose two-hundred dollars. Hang up.

Don't buy from an unfamiliar company. Ask and wait for any written material about them. And don't stop there. Check them out on line and with the Better Business Bureau or National Fraud Information Center. Get the salesperson's name, business identity, phone number and street and mailing address. (If the person doesn't want to share this information that will be a big clue that you're dealing with a con artist.)

Also, if you're considering giving to a charity that's new to you, don't pledge money without first checking out the organization to make sure it's legit. Do some research and find out how much of your charitable dollars get eaten up by high salaries and administration costs.

Don't pay for a free prize. If the caller tells you the payment is for taxes owed, that person is violating federal law.

If you're paying for services, don't pay in advance. I still remember my father paying a man in advance to fix the leaking bellows on our vintage player piano. The man never did fix them and the poor thing never did work well.

If you're entering the dating pool, get a second opinion on all candidates for your heart. Have a family member or cynical friend be your sounding board. If that person you met on It's Never too Late for Love.com is suddenly in need of a small loan, say "Adios" and move on to the next potential true love. If someone looks like a potential romantic partner, make sure you introduce that person to your family early on and make sure you meet his or her family and friends as well. Someone with neither family nor friends for you to meet should automatically be suspect.

Do remember that old phrase we've all heard: if it sounds too good to be true it probably is.

Don't allow family members with sketchy finances to run to the bank for you or make purchases. (Clue: if they're living with you their finances are sketchy.) In fact, don't rush to take in family members who are experiencing financial difficulties. And, if helping someone who is struggling with money management, relationship or substance abuse issues, set boundaries on how much financial assistance you will give. Any well can get drained, no matter how deep. You are no exception.

Finally, surround yourself with a good support team: a trusted family member with a proven moral compass that's in good working order, a good lawyer, accountant and money manager. Make sure you have wise people in your life who you can consult, use as sounding boards and as first lines of defense against predators.

1. Fbi.gov, *Scams and Safety, Common Fraud Schemes, Fraud Against Seniors,*

HTTPS://WWW.FBI.GOV/SCAMS-AND-SAFETY/COMMON-FRAUD-SCHEMES/SENIORS

1. Fbi.gov, *Sweetheart Scams*, Feb 9, 2012.

https://www.fbi.gov/audio-repository/news-podcasts-inside-sweetheart-scams.mp3/view

1. Long Roofing, *4 Signs You're Falling for a Roofing Scam*, Copyright 2019.

https://longroofing.com/blog/4-signs-youre-falling-roofing-scam/

1. ABC 30 action news, *3 Arrested for Allegedly Collecting Donations for Funeral of Boy Who Wasn't Dead*, September 20, 2018. https://abc30.com/3-arrested-for-funeral-fund-scam-that-included-photos-of-boy/4294386/
2. Identitytheftjournal.com: *The Most Common Causes of Identity Theft and How to Protect Yourself*, Copyright 2019.

http://www.identitytheftjournal.com/common-causes-identity-theft/

11. BEFORE THE CURTAIN IS PULLED

Death. None of us likes dealing with it or even talking about it, especially when it's our own. But we need to revisit this topic one last time so we can be prepared for that moment when our story here on earth ends and the final curtain falls.

You may be totally organized and have done everything you need to do to assure a smooth transition from this life to the after-life. If you have, you've got my permission to skip this chapter.

If you haven't, that could be for a number of reasons. According to attorney Richard C. Tizzano, author of the book *Accidental Safari* (an excellent book, by the way), there are three reasons why we put off dealing with these important details: denial, procrastination and apathy. Denial doesn't change the facts though. Procrastination leads to complications and regrets down the road. And apathy gets us nowhere. According to Mr. Tizzano, apathy is why fewer than fifty percent of us have executed a Last Will and Testament.[1] We don't want to be part of that particular statistic, so let me offer some suggestions to get you started.

The business of death is a complicated one and constantly changing, so the facts and anecdotes I'm sharing now may not apply two years from now or even one. This, of course, is why it's good to consult estate planning experts when deciding how your assets will be dispersed after you're gone.

Of course, you don't have to wait until after your death to give something to your heirs. If you have adult children who are paying off houses or college loans or need a new car, you might want to help them out now while you're around to enjoy seeing them improve their lives thanks to your generosity. So, let's take a quick side trip and talk about gifting money now rather than later.

As of this writing you can gift up to $15,000 each year per person to anyone, including family members without having to report it to the IRS and pay gift tax.[2] If you're married, as a couple you can give up to $28,000 ($14,000 from each of you) to an unlimited number of people each year without incurring a tax liability. (And why we should have to pay taxes on our own generosity will forever remain a mystery to me!) If you do give more than fifteen K to any one person during the tax year then you'll have to report it to your Uncle Sam on his Tax Form 709, "United States Gift (and Generation-Skipping Transfer) Tax Return." But you still won't have to pay taxes on the gift if it falls within the lifetime limit of tax-free gifts. (Isn't that kind of dear Uncle?) As of this writing, you are allowed to gift up to $5.6 million tax-free during your lifetime to family, friends or whomever.[3] Married couples can give almost $11 million away in their lifetime.[4] So, probably most of us won't have tax issues when it comes to our giving. If this just made your eyes glaze over, I encourage you to get expert financial help.

Let me also put a bug in your ear regarding the timing of your generosity. If you're planning on dumping your assets before you need to go in a nursing home and possibly throwing yourself on the mercy of Uncle Sam, be aware that, as of this writing, Medicaid investigates your finances back as far as five years. If it looks like you've been gifting money to get into a facility using Medicaid Uncle will take those resources back.

Another important question to ask yourself – do you want a will or do you want to set up a revocable living trust? There's a big difference between the two.

A trust will save your heirs from dealing with probate. There are two types of trusts: irrevocable and revocable. Most people don't opt for an irrevocable trust because it involves turning over ownership of your property to the trust and its trustees permanently A revocable trust can be changed and isn't necessarily permanent. The beauty of a trust is that it doesn't require probate, the court supervised process that's required if you have a will. (Many people prefer to avoid probate because it delays the distribution of their assets. Also, with a will, everything you're doing becomes a matter of public record.) With a trust your successor trustee can step in if you reach a point where you can't manage your own affairs. These are complicated animals and nothing you want to tackle on your own.

If you've earned your living in the arts, say as an author or songwriter, this adds another wrinkle. Your copyrights keep going long after you're gone. If you still have work out there for sale, any royalties you earned during your lifetime continue after death. Make sure you've jumped through the proper hoops to assign those royalties to someone. Again, consulting a lawyer would be wise.

Whether your assets are few and your wishes simple or you have several properties and/or investments it really does behoove you to consult an elder law attorney who can ensure that what you leave behind will get dispersed according to your wishes. Ask around, do your research. Find someone who comes highly recommended and get going on this.

It's a good idea to discuss ahead of time who will inherit what. Decide and explain how you are going to divide those family treasures. Will the child who foots the bill for your care inherit the house? If so, make sure everyone knows this and get it all in writing so there's no fighting after you're gone. Find out who wants

Grandma's crystal, who's going to get Dad's signed baseball, and who wants that special picture hanging in the hall. One afternoon in my mother's later years, we spent some time talking about who she'd like to receive various pieces of her china, furniture, and home décor. I made notes and taped slips of paper underneath and to the backs of many items so there'd be no confusion when the time came. For my own kids, I put together a list to email to both of them listing who gets what. After they had a chance to look it over I made any necessary changes, then listed the various sentimental treasures in a document and sent it to both of them. This way there will be no confusion and both children and grandchildren will be assured of having something that was in the family.

Like money, some family treasures can be gifted while you're alive. That way you can have the pleasure of seeing your children enjoying them. Want to downsize to a smaller Christmas tree? How about having a pre-Christmas family party and letting the kids chose favorite ornaments to use on their trees? Let them draw numbers and take turns. That way you won't be playing favorites. You can do the same thing with anything from jewelry to serving dishes.

You're probably not going to get rid of everything, however. So if you're worried your kids will end up fighting over who gets the Limoges chocolate pot or the painting that hung in the hall, then put those in a codicil. For less valuable items it's a good idea to state in the will that you will leave a letter or list designating what goes to whom. Make a memorandum and have it with you when you go to see your lawyer. It needs to be in existence before the will is signed so there can be no suspicion of it having been changed after your will has been made. Hopefully, you would keep this list with your will. But I think it's also a good idea to make sure your heirs all have a copy ahead of time.

In researching this I read that extreme detail in a will can attract unwelcome IRS attention. So, rather than listing your possessions in detail you might simply want to write in your will "my tangible personal property" and outline how your heirs should divvy it up. In our case, our son will be handling the sale of property and I'm assigning my daughter to distribute all household items that haven't already been promised to the other women in the family as she sees fit.

There's more to getting prepared for death than simply having a will. If you're naming one of your children as executor of your will, it's a good idea to have that child's name on your checking account so necessary bills can be paid after you're gone. I have a friend right now who's gnawing off her arm in frustration because her mother made no such arrangements. Mom still had outstanding bills and owed money on her house, but her assets are trapped in probate and her daughter, who is the executor of her will, has no way to pay the bills.

Also, make sure that you have assigned power of attorney to someone you trust and that you have an advance directive (living will). Also, tell your family what you want so there will be no bickering at the death bed. You will take so much emotional pressure off your kids if you've made your wishes known concerning those end of life scenarios.

Ideally, we don't want to leave a rat's nest behind for our kids to deal with when we depart this world. If we can make sure things are taken care of legally it will make life easier for all concerned.

The same applies to our mates. So many things we take for granted, things like joint accounts and credit cards. But problems can come up with them after a spouse dies.

A week after my brother died, my sister-in-law went to Costco to get gas and discovered her credit card no longer worked. The account had been closed. Her name was on the card along with my brother's but he had taken out the card. His name was the primary name on it, and on his death the account was closed.

Needless to say, this was the last thing she needed on top of dealing with the shock of losing her husband.

Sooo, do you and your spouse both have a credit card in your own name? And how about bank accounts? Whose name is on them?

Bank accounts are the tip of the iceberg. Here's a check list of things you need to attend to:

Make sure you've designated an heir for any stocks or bonds you might own and that this is in the will.

Know where your marriage license is. You'll need this when you apply for survivor's benefits.

Know your spouse's social security number and make sure your spouse knows yours.

Know where your will is. Is it in a safe place? Does whoever you've named the executor of your will know where it is?

Do you have a safe deposit box? A post office box? Does the executor of your will have a key to each of them?

Does the executor of your will have a key to your house/condo/summer place?

If you have a pet that could outlive you, have you asked someone to take it after you're gone? (Don't leave Pete the parrot out in the cold!)

As to final resting places, have you made arrangements? Does your family know your final wishes? Burial or cremation? Open casket or closed? Do you have burial plots already purchased? Have you pre-paid your cremation? Is that information easily accessible to your family?

Earlier we talked about deciding how we want to remember our loved ones. It's also important, if you have certain wishes about how you'd like to be remembered to let them be known. Do you want a funeral or celebration of life? If you do, what songs do you want played? What pictures do you want displayed? And is there something special you want mentioned in your obituary? (You might consider actually writing it yourself ahead of time. After all, no one knows your life as well as you.) Would you love to have people make donations to a certain charity in your name? Don't leave your family guessing. It's best if you have a file with all vital information in one handy place that addresses all these issues.

The more things we can take care of ahead of time the more stress we'll remove from our loved one's shoulders.

Speaking of stress, have you gone through the painful exercise of having to sort through your deceased parents' possessions? It can be daunting and emotionally draining, not to mention time-consuming. Chances are, when you depart this world your children will still be very busy living in it – perhaps still working, involved with their own children and grandchildren, so please resist the temptation to hold onto all those doodads and unnecessary paperwork you've been collecting for years.

I wish I could say we've done this. I've already apologized in advance several times to our kids for all the stuff they're going to have to wade through.

Don't be like us! Reduce the amount of flotsam and jetsam kicking around. Shred those old documents. Lose the broken jewelry, outdated technology, clothes you no longer wear, extra plastic bags and expired medicine and food items. Unless, of course, you're upset with your kids. Then punish the little buzzards and keep it all. And trust me, making them comb through all that excess junk will be punishment.

Again, I know we don't like thinking about the fact that we're mortal, especially when we're healthy and having fun. But nobody gets off this planet alive. Your time will come. Deal with these details now and then you can skip back to the dance floor or return to that good book you were reading and not have to think about this again. (Unless you sell the house or the boat. Or buy a house or a boat. Then remember to prove to your loved ones that you, indeed, love them and update your will.) All right. Enough said about that.

Now, let's talk about another important thing you might want to leave your family: the gift of family history. Are your kids starting to ask questions about the different branches of the family tree or why you always put nutmeg in your meatloaf? Perhaps it's time to sit down and talk about your life. Even if you feel like you can't get around much anymore or do all the things you used to be able to, this is something you can do.

At some point most of us have questions about where we came from, what life was like for our parents growing up or raising kids. We find ourselves asking, "Did my mom ever feel like this?"

Sometimes, by the time we get around to asking those questions Mom isn't around anymore and it's too late to know. A gift of your memories put in writing or recorded is one of the best legacies you can leave your children.

You may think your life isn't all that interesting, but I bet it's more interesting than you realize. You probably have some funny stories of things that happened in your family when you were growing up or when your kids were small. Or before you even had kids.

I remember enjoying looking at a picture of my dad when he was young and singing in a department store quartet. My mom also had a picture that had been taken of the two of them when he was Santa for some community event. She was standing behind him, giving him a hug and hiding her baby bump. It was a cute picture and fun to learn the secret behind the pose.

Even more entertaining than these pictures were the many crazy tales my father would tell of his life growing up. It was a wild one and Dad did everything from running away with the circus to trying his hand at being a bootlegger. He changed once he met my mom and became a pillar of the community, but to my brothers and me (and later the grandkids) that time of his life

wasn't half as fascinating as all the crazy stuff that .
him before he settled down.

Further up my family tree we find robbers, one of w.
claimed to have found gold buried in the back yard. This
announcement was followed by, "Load up the wagon. We're leaving tonight." It is strongly suspected he didn't find that gold in the back yard. My father is long gone, but my family still enjoys sharing these family stories.

My mother-in-law, a feisty Aussie who came to America on the last war bride ship, lived an equally colorful life and I used to love to listen to her talk about the many ups and downs she experienced.

What stories about your life growing up do you have to share? Did your family survive tough times financially? Did you grow up on a farm? Start your own business? Win consecutive blue ribbons at the county fair? Juggle multiple admirers? What was work like for you? What was your first big purchase as an adult, as a married couple? What about that first baby? Any off-to-have-baby stories to share? What was your first job? Your first car? What appliances, tools, and toys did you grow up using that are now obsolete? Inquiring minds probably at some point will want to know.

The idea of writing about your life might feel intimidating. You're not alone. People fear writing almost as much as they fear public speaking. You might be good with numbers or a smashing business success, but the idea of having to put words on paper terrifies you. Don't worry if writing is not in your wheelhouse. Don't worry about looking foolish because your grammar isn't perfect. Your descendants aren't going to care about that. What they are going to care about is having some sort of record of your life.

So, where to begin? Start by thinking about how you'd like to proceed. Do you want to write about your whole life or is there one particular time that feels more interesting? If you're summarizing your whole life you're writing a biography. If you're writing about a particular time then you're writing a memoir.

Whatever you decide to write, it will be appreciated by the following generations. Your personal story brings history alive in a way that a textbook can never do.

Years ago I interviewed my mother-in-law for a book. A while later my husband and I interviewed her again, this time with my father-in-law, and we filmed it. My interview with her concentrated primarily on the years before she met my father-in-law when she was dealing with the fallout from having married an abusive husband, but she also gave me snapshot glimpses into her life as a child. One particular scene that stuck with me was one that took place during the Great Depression in the thirties. I had always thought this economic slump only hit America, so was surprised to learn that wasn't the case. Australia had its struggles as well and so did her family. She talked about the uncle who lived with them trying desperately to find work, getting discouraged and then getting drunk, and how she and her cousins hid under one of the beds when he'd come home in a violent mood. A glimpse into her childhood and a story about her first marriage, then some reminiscences of the early years of her marriage with my father-in-law – it wasn't a daily record, but she hit the highlights, the most interesting reminiscences. We learned that he went AWOL to marry her and they spent their wedding night on the beach. (That sounded really romantic until she talked about the wharf rat nibbling on her hair!) I didn't need every minute of her whole life. The highlights were enough.

It will be the same with your loved ones. If you're writing your life story, keep in mind the fact that you don't have to cover every moment. You don't necessarily need to begin with your birth (unless the doctor didn't think you'd survive), and you don't have to list every birthday you had and what you did to celebrate (unless your parents gave you a hundred shares of blue-chip stock that was the foundation for the family fortune. Hit the interesting highlights. Were you a star quarterback? Did you save your best friend in the jungles of Vietnam? Or did your best friend save you and that's why you're here today? Did you launch a business? Lose a business? If so, what happened?

If you don't want to write about your whole life you can go the memoir route and recount what you feel to be the most interesting time of your life. Perhaps you could write about how you built your business. Or how you met your other half. Maybe you want to simply write down some of the funny things that happened to you growing up. Or maybe your family tree is as twisted and crazy as mine and you want to write down a few of those family legends before they get lost in the mists of time. That's good stuff, too.

Have I intimidated you yet? Don't pull your hair and run screaming into the night. I have some suggestions for how you might want to tackle such a project.

First of all, decide whether you want to write a biography or a memoir. If it's a biography, divide your life into sections: Childhood, Young Love or Teen Years and Adulthood. That way you'll have an idea where to place your various stories. As you reminisce, get in touch with your inner reporter and interview yourself. Be sure to ask yourself how you felt about different things that happened to you. How did the current events of your time affect your life? What decisions are you proud of? Did you make choices you regret? If you could live your life over what would you do differently?

If you're writing a memoir, a lot of those same questions will apply. You'll simply be focusing in on a specific time and adventure.

Such a big job can feel daunting, so break it into smaller jobs that you can peck away at. And don't stress over deadlines. You didn't live your life overnight. You won't be able to write about it overnight, either.

As you're working through your story have someone in your

family read it and give you feedback. What didn't that person understand? Were certain cultural references unclear? Getting this kind of input as you move along will ensure clarity.

If you feel you don't have a gift for writing and don't want to tackle it, consider hiring someone to write your story for you. Get thee to the internet and type in biography writers and a plethora of services will pop up. Your local librarian or chamber of commerce might also be able to recommend someone.

Or buy one of those memory journals filled with questions where all you have to do is fill in the blanks.

I purchased one of these for my own mother and she filled out some of it, but many of those questions were left blank. I now wish I'd encouraged her to write more in it. Ah, well. I'm glad for what I have. Chances are, even if they don't seem interested now, after you're gone your family will also be interested.

You might feel more comfortable simply talking. Turn on your phone or video camera and start reminiscing. Or, better yet, get a family member to interview you and record it so you'll feel like you're simply having a conversation. That can prevent you from getting camera shy.

Another thing to consider is going through old photos and making sure you've made notes on the back about the people in the pictures. Two or three generations down the road, someone looking at them will appreciate the fact that you pointed out which person was you and which person was Aunt Hattie. And, by the way, you don't need to save every picture you ever took. Sort through and find the ones that tell a story or answer a family history question. Pass on pictures to your children and grandchildren that tell their personal history. If possible, collect them in photo albums or have them scanned and put on a disc. There are a number of companies who offer this service and it's a good way to streamline those memory treasures and get rid of some of the excess stuff kicking around the house.

All the things I've suggested in this chapter, taken together, probably look like a very daunting to-do list. I suggest you turn them into exactly that. List the things you need to do in order of importance and work your way through at a pace that's comfortable for you. Starting early on these final details when there is no emergency and no urgency will save you a lot of grief down the road.

1. Richard C. Tizzano, *Accidental Safari*, (Richard C. Tizzano, 2017).
2. Smartasset.com: *Gift Tax Limit 2018: How Much Can You Gift?*, Copyright 2018.

HTTPS://SMARTASSET.COM/RETIREMENT/GIFT-TAX-LIMITS

1. Forbes.com: *IRS Announces 2018 Estate and Gift Tax Limits.*

https://www.forbes.com/sites/ashleaebeling/2017/10/19/irs-announces-2018-estate-and-gift-tax-limits-11-2-million-per-couple/#449a2d14a4b8

1. Mlrp.co: *IRS Increases Annual Gift Tax Exclusion for 2018*, Copyright 2018.

https://www.mlrpc.com/articles/irs-increases-annual-gift-tax-exclusion-

1. Aarp.org: *Half of Adults Do Not Have Wills*, Copyright 2017.

https://www.aarp.org/money/investing/info-2017/half-of-adults-do-not-have-wills.html

12. ENCOURAGING WORDS

Aging is not for sissies, it's true, and if you're still struggling with the reality of where you are and wishing you could travel back in time, well, I hear you. I keep thinking, fifty would be good. But then I think of the hard things I had to go through after fifty and realize I don't want to repeat them.

Not that going back is an option. This story only goes forward. That being the case, isn't it worth our while to each keep on writing the best story we can?

I'm still working away at mine and I'm grateful for every day I have left to do it. I want to make my story better, and I'm determined to make the most of the years I have left here on Planet Earth.

I hope you are, too. So let me leave you with some quotes and final words of wisdom that I hope will encourage you to keep writing your own unique life story.

"Aging is an extraordinary process where you become the person you always should have been."

– David Bowie

. . .

"Is not wisdom found among the aged? Does not long life bring understanding?"

– Job 12:12, the Bible, New International Version

"Aging is not 'lost youth' but a new stage of opportunity and strength."

– Betty Friedan

"Youth is the gift of nature, but age is a work of art."

– Polish poet Stanislaw Jerzy Lec

"Age is something that doesn't matter, unless you are a cheese."

– Luis Buñuel, film maker

"There is a fountain of youth: it is your mind, your talents, the creativity you bring to your life and the lives of people you love. When you learn to tap this source, you will truly have defeated age."

– Sophia Loren

"Gray hair is a crown of splendor ..."

– Proverbs16:31, the Bible, New International Version

"Age wrinkles the body. Quitting wrinkles the soul."

– Douglas MacArthur

. . .

"Age is an issue of mind over matter. If you don't mind, it doesn't matter."

– Mark Twain

Know that you are the perfect age. Each year is special and precious, for you shall only live it once. Be comfortable with growing older."

– author Louise Hay

"Those who love deeply never grow old; they may die of old age, but they die young."

– Ben Franklin

"Getting old is like climbing a mountain; you get a little out of breath, but the view is much better!"

– Ingrid Bergman

None are so old as those who have outlived enthusiasm."

– Henry David Thoreau

"Count your age by friends, not years. Count your life by smiles, not tears."

– John Lennon

"The righteous will flourish like a palm tree, they will grow like a cedar of Lebanon; planted in the house of the Lord, they will flourish in the courts of our God. They will still bear fruit in old age, they will still stay fresh and green, proclaiming, 'The Lord is upright; he is my Rock and there is no wickedness in him.'"

– the Bible, Psalm 92: 12-15, New International Version

How's that for a great collection of inspiring words?

You might be in a place right now where your life isn't perfect. It's harder to hide from those aches and pains as we get older. We deal with health issues and often heart issues of loss and sorrow, but as long as we're still here dealing, we're still in the game.

Let me leave you with one final quote:

"There are six myths about old age: 1. That it's a disease, a disaster. 2. That we are mindless. 3. That we are sexless. 4. That we are useless. 5. That we are powerless. 6. That we are all alike."

—Maggie Kuhn, founder of the Gray Panthers movement

WE'RE NOT useless and we don't have to be hopeless. Let's dispel those myths. Old is not a four-letter word. Don't let anyone tell you any different.

ACKNOWLEDGMENTS

Before we begin, allow me a moment to thank all the people who so kindly shared their expertise and contributed their advice on various topics covered in this book. I'm especially indebted to Peggy Doviak, financial planner extraordinaire, for allowing me to pick her brain, to Paula Eykelhof, friend and former editor for her input and suggestions, to Ruth Ross, who served as my editor on this project, and to Ellen Johnson and my wonderful husband for serving as first readers.